HYPERBARIC OXYGENATION

Publication Number 640

AMERICAN LECTURE SERIES®

A Monograph in
AMERICAN LECTURES IN ANESTHESIOLOGY

Edited by

JOHN ADRIANI, M.D.
Director, Department of Anesthesia
Charity Hospital of Louisiana
New Orleans, Louisiana

HYPERBARIC OXYGENATION

By

CHARLES B. PITTINGER, M.D.

Professor and Chairman, Department of Anesthesiology
Associate Professor, Department of Pharmacology
Vanderbilt University School of Medicine
Anesthesiologist-in-Chief, Vanderbilt University Hospital
Consultant in Anesthesia, Veterans Administration Hospital
Nashville, Tennessee

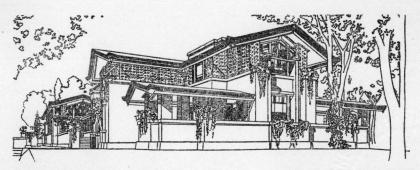

CHARLES C THOMAS · PUBLISHER
Springfield · Illinois · U.S.A.

Published and Distributed Throughout the World by
CHARLES C THOMAS • PUBLISHER
BANNERSTONE HOUSE
301-327 East Lawrence Avenue, Springfield, Illinois, U.S.A.
NATCHEZ PLANTATION HOUSE
735 North Atlantic Boulevard, Fort Lauderdale, Florida, U.S.A.

© *1966, by* CHARLES C THOMAS • PUBLISHER
Library of Congress Catalog Card Number: 66-12447

With THOMAS BOOKS careful attention is given to all details of manufacturing and design. It is the Publisher's desire to present books that are satisfactory as to their physical qualities and artistic possibilities and appropriate for their particular use. THOMAS BOOKS will be true to those laws of quality that assure a good name and good will.

Printed in the United States of America
N-1

DEDICATION

*To my wife, Gertrude, and our
children, Suzanne, Charley and Katy*

Preface

THIS MONOGRAPH HAS been prepared to provide a concise introduction to the various aspects of hyperbaric oxygenation. The scope is broad in order to satisfy diversified interests and to provide to each a balanced view of the basic scientific and clinical implications of the subject.

Four categories of readers were considered: (1) those desiring merely a conversational acquaintance with the currently popular subject; (2) those with research inclinations voluntarily committed to its laboratory or clinical investigation; (3) clinicians, who perforce are confronted with its application or problems associated with it; (4) students for whom the subject deserves to be a part of a progressive medical education.

The information offered has been culled from widely scattered sources and compiled to provide a concise insight to the history, theory, scientific investigation and clinical application of hyperbaric oxygenation, and appreciation of the attendant problems and complexities.

A broad survey of a subject which offers neither suggestions for progressive reading nor escape from the subjective interpretation of the author would be of limited value. To circumvent such limitations and to extend the practicality of the monograph, selected references are provided for those who wish to pursue various phases in depth. The comprehensiveness of the bibliographies was intentional in an effort to provide within a single volume references to the scattered sources of pertinent information. Such further pursuit is essential for intelligent experimentation or clinical application of hyperbaric oxygenation. Since the monograph is not a manual of procedures, those seeking such direction will also find the bibliographies helpful.

The author is grateful to John Adriani, M.D., Director, Department of Anesthesiology, Charity Hospital, New Orleans, for his invitation to prepare the manuscript and his efforts in editing it. An expression of appreciation is extended to Mr. Raymond Snyder of the Ingersall Research Center, Borg-Warner Corporation, Des Plaines, Illinois, and to Dr. Jack Van Elk, Section of Cardiology, Lutheran General Hospital, Park Ridge, Illinois, for courtesies associated with a visit to the hyperbaric facility at the latter institution. To Miss Eleanor Steinke, Director of the Medical Library of Vanderbilt University School of Medicine and to her staff, the author is indebted for their courteous and proficient assistance. To Mrs. Ann Starkey, particular thanks are due for her stenographic services.

C. B. P.

Contents

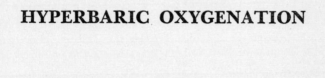

HYPERBARIC OXYGENATION

1

Historical Development

H YPERBARIC OXYGENATION (H.O.) is oxygen therapy applied within a pressure chamber under circumstances which provide alveolar partial pressures of the gas exceeding those possible from the inhalation of pure oxygen at atmospheric pressure. The resultant hyperoxemia is intermediate in the production of elevations in tissue tensions of oxygen. The objective of the therapeutic regimen is the development of elevated tensions of the gas within mitochondria, the presumed site of its most significant cellular activity.

Current medical interest in H.O. originated with the encouraging report of Churchill-Davidson and his associates[10] in 1955 pertaining to its application in radiotherapy and that of Boerema and coworkers[7] in 1956 regarding its use as an adjunct to cardiac surgery. Interest was enhanced subsequently by the dramatic demonstration by Boerema[8] of the possibility of sustaining life in a bloodless pig perfused with saline solution while the animal breathed oxygen at three atmospheres absolute.

The designation of pressure in terms of atmospheres absolute represents conventional hyperbaric terminology. Its consistent use in relation to H.O. is urged to avoid ambiguity. Ambient pressure at sea level is regarded as one atmosphere absolute, or approximately fifteen pounds per square inch (15 psi). Gauges designed to measure pressures above atmospheric indicate ambient pressure as zero. Thus a registered pressure of 1 atmosphere or 15 psi on a gauge represents 2 atmospheres absolute; one of 2 atmospheres or 30 psi is equivalent to 3 atmospheres absolute, etc.

Technical advances of modern engineering have afforded a variety of pressure chambers with almost unlimited degrees of sophistication. Large facilities for H.O. exist at Lutheran General Hospital, Park Ridge, Ill., Duke University, Durham, N. C., Children's Hospital, Boston, Mass., The Mount Sinai Hospital, N. Y. C., and Minneapolis General Hospital Research Foundation, Inc.,

Minneapolis, Minn., in this country; in Europe such exist at the Wilhelmina Gasthuis, Amsterdam and Leiden University in Holland, and at the Royal Infirmary, Glasgow, Scotland. Numerous commercially available units of smaller size are in use or on order in the United States.

Technical developments are in advance of the basic scientific knowledge required for safe and judicious application of H.O. Recognition of the need for a scientific approach in its applications is manifested in the 1963 report of the Ad Hoc Committee on Hyperbaric Oxygenation of the Division of Medical Sciences of the National Academy of Sciences and was evident at the 1964 Conference on H.O. sponsored jointly by the New York Academy of Sciences and the National Academy of Sciences. Whereas the concerted efforts of various scientific disciplines to foster such an approach would favor fruitful development of H.O., imprudent and unscientific applications of it on the part of individual enthusiasts could lead to its abandonment.

H.O. is not an achievement of the past decade; rather, its present status reflects developments and hindrances during hundreds of years. Its developmental history is not only interesting, but also rewarding in the information provided. It begins in the distant past with man's initial exposure to hyperbaric conditions through diving in quest for food, treasures, escape or pleasure. Eventually, his scientific curiosity led to experimentation aimed toward allowing him longer periods of submergence. Breathing of pressurized air by divers submerged within an inverted metal vessel was mentioned by Aristotle (384-322 B.C.). An exhibition of such a fete was held in 1538 at Toledo, Spain. In 1797, Klingert invented a diving gear consisting of a metallic cylinder which encased the body from head to hips and subsequently improved it by the addition of an air supply for breathing. Siebe, in 1819, devised a diving apparatus which incorporated a metal helmet into which air was pumped. Subsequent refinements led to the modern diving suit provided with a constant flow of compressed air breathed at a pressure proportional to depth of submersion.

In 1841, Triger[25] reported the use of the first caisson for submarine mining operations. This initiated the simultaneous exposure of more than one person to hyperbaric conditions within a single apparatus.

Accidents and illnesses associated with increasing exposures of persons to elevated pressures eventually caused a focusing of attention upon the physiologic aspects of hyperbaricity. The first to do so in a detailed scientific study was Paul Bert whose monumental compilation, La Pression Barometrique,[4] is fortunately available in an excellent English translation.[5] Therein are contained observations of phenomena related to the operation of hyperbaric chambers, such as convulsive and pulmonary disorders associated with oxygen toxicity, lethargy and disorientation now attributed to nitrogen narcosis and gas embolism occurring with decompression. Heller and associates[15] compiled a comprehensive treatise on caisson disease in 1900.

The studies of gas solubility and embolism by Haldane were the basis for the establishment of safety rules regulating decompression rates adopted by the British Admiralty in 1907 to minimize decompression sickness. A review of his many researches was published in a monograph[14] on respiration.

The U. S. Navy has fostered extensive physiologic researches in the interest of diving safety. The contributions of Behnke and his associates in their investigations of decompression sickness, oxygen toxicity and nitrogen narcosis will be discussed in subsequent chapters.

Extensive bibliographical references to pertinent information including early therapeutic efforts have been prepared by Hoff and Greenbaum.[17,18] The U. S. Navy Diving Manual[26] is a valuable directive of decompression procedures which is advised in the operation of pressure chambers.

The first suggestion of the clinical application of variations of air pressure is accredited to Henshaw[16] in England who postulated in 1664 the benefits of compression in the treatment of acute diseases and rarification for chronic disorders. For that purpose he designed a chamber called a domicilium for raising and lowering pressure. In 1783, the Haarlem Academy of Science in Holland offered a prize, never claimed, for the design of a pressure chamber for therapeutic use. It was not until 1834 that Junod[19] described and built the first such chamber to investigate the physiological and therapeutic effects of increased and decreased air pressures. His chamber was not well received because of its limited size and lack of control of pressure variations. Soon thereafter, Tabarie[23,24] investigated the effects of compression and rarification applied to the entire body, and incidentally also to all of the body except the head, thus simulating the effects of modern tank respirators. In his treatment of respiratory diseases within the chamber, he stressed slow changes in pressure. Concurrently, Pravas[21,22] employed compressed air "baths" in his orthopedic clinic at Lyons, instituted therapy for tuberculosis, and eventually established treatments of up to a dozen persons simultaneously in a large chamber. His reports, though not medically convincing, stimulated the development of health spas offering similar treatment. This movement was aided by Bertin's outline[6] of the history and clinical indications for use of pressure chambers.

During the latter half of the 19th century, Europe was dotted with numerous pressure treatment centers including those operated by Milliet at Lyons and Nice, Grindrod in England, von Vivenot in Vienna, Sandahl in Stockholm, von Liebig in Baden-Baden and Hovent in Brussels. The enthusiastic, empirical movement was spurred in 1887 by Arntzenius' publication[2] of *De Pneumatische Therapie* with some 300 references on the subject.

During the last quarter of the eighteenth century in Europe, another type of inhalation therapy was emerging as a result of the discoveries of carbon dioxide, nitrous oxide, carbon monoxide, hydrogen and oxygen. Though initially the interest of pneumatic chemists, these gases quickly attracted the attention of physicians. Such was the case with oxygen which had been discovered independently by Scheele in 1772 and Priestley in 1774. The story is interestingly related by Cartwright[9] of the biological interests of Priestley, Lavoisier and Davy and the development of the famous Pneumatic Institution at Bristol by Thomas Beddoes, a physician, and his associate, James Watt, an engineer. Apparently, with good intentions, excessive credulity, and an irresistible urge to publish inconclusive data, Beddoes administered the above gases for therapeutic purposes. Although accredited for initiating oxygen therapy, he failed to establish it upon sound scientific principles. The reason for the failure of the Pneumatic Institution is apparent from the report[3] of its operation in 1795.

With the increasing availability of oxygen, its use spread through Europe, including centers possessing hyperbaric chambers. How extensively the gas was employed in hyperbaric therapy is not clear. There is no evidence that partial pressures of oxygen such as those now in vogue were regularly employed prior to the current interest in H.O.

On this continent, possibly because of its remoteness from the above sites of activity, lesser inclinations toward experimental techniques, or lack of conviction of the benefits reported from abroad, few physicians were caught in the early enthusiasm of hyperbaric therapy. Nevertheless, reference to pneumatic chambers in Toronto, Rochester and Buffalo were made by Lee[20] in 1867. Ethridge[13] published on the subject in 1873. Corning[12] employed compressed air in his practice in New York at the turn of the century. The transient operations in the 1920's of a chamber by Cunningham at Kansas City, and the elaborate facility at Cleveland are matters of regrettable record.[1,11]

The inappropriateness of enthusiastic empiricism as an approach to the establishment of a therapeutic regimen is well documented. The dangers and disappointments associated with the misuse of a technique are prone to result in deprivation of its possible benefits. Such has been the previous fate of hyperbaric therapy imprudently applied in the treatment of: amenorrhea, anemia, anorexia, aortic stenosis, aphonia, asthma, atelectasis, bronchiectasis, bronchitis, catarrh, chlorosis, chorea, conjunctivitis, deafness, diabetes, eczema, emphysema, hemoptysis, hysteria, irregular menstruation, kyphosis, laryngeal and tracheal stenosis, laryngitis, leucorrhea, menorrhagia, mitral insufficiency, neuralgia, otorrhea, pleurisy, post-influenzal depression, smallpox, syphilis, tuberculosis, viper bites and whooping cough!

H.O. is currently being investigated in areas where theoretical considerations suggest possible benefits. Included among those are radiotherapy of cancer, temporary vascular occlusion during surgery, vascular insufficiencies from other causes, anaerobic and other infections, carbon monoxide and barbiturate poisonings, infant resuscitation, shock and hyaline membrane disease.

In succeeding chapters, the theoretical bases for these applications will be provided along with an indication of their progresses. The eventual security of appropriate H.O. among acceptable medical techniques will be dependent upon the predominance of scientific methodology over reckless empiricism and the avoidance of foibles and faddism in experimental applications.

References

1. A.M.A. Bureau of Investigation: The Cunningham "Tank Treatment". The alleged value of compressed air in the treatment of diabetes mellitus, pernicious anemia and carcinoma. *J.A.M.A., 90:*1494, 1928.

2. Arntzenius, A. K. W.: *De Pneumatische Therapie.* Amsterdam, Sheltema and Holkema's Boekhandel, 1887.

3. Beddoes, T., and Watt, J.: *Considerations on the Medicinal Use and on the Production of Factitious Airs.* Bristol, 1795.

4. Bert, P.: *La Pression Barometrique.* Paris, Masson, 1878.

5. Bert, P.: *Barometric Pressure.* Translation by M. A. and F. A. Hitchcock. Columbus, College Book, 1943.

6. Bertin, E.: *Étude clinique de l'emploi et des effets du bain d'air comprimé dans le traitement de diverses maladies.* Paris, Bailliére, 1855.

7. Boerema, I., Kroll, J. A., Meijne, N. G., Lokin, E., Kroon, B., and Huiskes, J. W.: High atmospheric pressure as an aid to cardiac surgery. *Arch. Chir. Neerl., 8:*193, 1956.

8. Boerema, I., Meijne, N. G., Brummelkamp, W. K., Bouma, S., Mensch, M. H., Kamerans, F., Hanf, S. M., and Aalderen, W. Van: Life without blood. *J. Cardiov. Surg., 1:*133, 1960.

9. Cartwright, F. F.: *The English Pioneers of Anaesthesia.* Bristol, Wright, 1952.

10. Churchill-Davidson, I., Sanger, C., and Thomlinson, R. H.: High pressure oxygen and radiotherapy. *Lancet, 1:*1091, 1955.

11. Cleveland Engineering: *21:*Cover and pp. 3-8 (Nov. 8), 1928.

12. Corning, J. L.: The use of compressed air in conjunction with medicinal solutions in the treatment of nervous and mental affections. *Med. Rec. N. Y., 40:*225, 1891.

13. Etheridge, J. H.: Compressed air. *Chicago Med. J., 30:*166, 1873.

14. Haldane, J. S.: *Respiration.* New Haven, Yale, 1922.

15. HELLER, R., MAGER, W., AND SCHRÖTTER: *Luftdruckerkrankungen mit besonderer Berücksichtigung der Sogenannten Caisson-krankeit*. Wien, Alfred Hölder, 1900.

16. HENSHAW, 1664 (England). See Simpson, A.: *Compressed Air as a Therapeutic Agent*. Edinburg, Sutherland and Knox, 1957.

17. HOFF, E. C.: *A Bibliographical Source-Book of Compressed Air, Diving and Submarine Medicine*. ONR, U. S. Govt. Printing Office, 1948.

18. HOFF, E. C., AND GREENBAUM, L. J.: *A Bibliographical Source-Book of Compressed Air and Submarine Medicine*. Vol. 2. ONR, U. S. Govt. Printing Office, 1954.

19. JUNOD, V. T.: Recherches physiologiques et thérapeutiques sur les effets de la compression et de raréfaction de l'air, tant sur le corps que sur les membres isolés. *Rev. Med. Franc Etrange, 3:* 350, 1834.

20. LEE, C. A.: Extract from a lecture on the physiological and remedial effects of increased pressure of the atmosphere. *Buffalo Med. Surg. J., 6:*199, 1867.

21. PRAVAS: Memoire sur l'application du bain d'air comprimé au traitement des affections tuberculeuses, des hemorrhagies capillaires et des surdités catarrholes. *Bull. Acad. Nat. Med., (Paris),* 2:985, 1837-38.

22. PRAVAS: Essai sur l'emploi médical de l'air comprimé. *C. R. Acad. Sci. (Paris), 34:*427, 1852.

23. TABARIÉ, E.: Recherches sur les effets des variations dans la pression atmospherique á la surgace due corps. *C. R. Acad. Sci. (Paris), 6:*896, 1838.

24. TABARIÉ, E.: Sur l'action therapeutique de l'air comprimé. *C. R. Acad. Sci. (Paris), 11:*26, 1840.

25. TRIGER, E: Memoire sur un appareil á air comprimé, pour le percement des puits de mines et autres travous, sous les laux et dans les sables submergés. *C. R. Acad. Sci. (Paris), 13:*884, 1841.

26. U. S. NAVY DIVING MANUAL. Dept. of the Navy, U. S. Govt. Printing Office, 1959.

2

Physiologic Considerations

THE FUNDAMENTAL PHYSIOLOGIC process of H.O. concerns the uptake of inspired oxygen and its cellular distribution via the blood stream. Since these events represent the goal of H.O. and the means of its achievement, an understanding of them is essential to an appreciation of their consequences.

H.O. involves quantities of dissolved oxygen in excess of those feasible at atmospheric pressure. Solution is affected through application of Henry's Law which states that the solubility of a gas at a given temperature is proportional to the pressure of the gas to which a liquid is exposed. In a mixture of gases, each component exerts a partial pressure dependent upon the relative number or percentage of its molecules present. The sum of the partial pressures of the various components equals the total pressure of the system; an increase in total pressure affects a proportionate increase in partial pressures. The solubility of each component is a function of its partial pressure and unrelated to the presence of the other gases. In H.O., the solubility of oxygen is augmented by increasing the percentage of the gas inhaled and raising the total pressure within a chamber.

The oxygen content of air is approximately 20.9 vols.%, representing a partial pressure of 158 mm Hg. Alveolar partial pressure of the gas is about 100 mm Hg which is reflected by a similar tension in arterial blood. The total oxygen content of the latter is 20 vols.%, or 20 ml per 100 ml of blood. Most of this oxygen is combined with hemoglobin which is about 97 per cent saturated. Only 0.3 ml of the gas is dissolved in the plasma. The supply of dissolved oxygen is normally replenished through reduction of oxyhemoglobin. This dissociation of oxyhemoglobin accounts for a saturation of hemoglobin to the extent of about 70 per cent in venous blood.

If pure oxygen is breathed, its alveolar partial pressure eventually reaches about 670 mm Hg which represents an almost seven-fold increase. The change is reflected in arterial blood where the total oxygen content is elevated to 22 vols.%. Since hemoglobin is normally almost saturated, complete saturation is reached by the uptake of only a small fraction of the additional amount. Most of the additional 2 ml of oxygen per 100 ml of arterial blood is present as dissolved gas. Further increases in the partial pressure of oxygen serve only to increase the amount in physical solution since hemoglobin is already completely saturated. Thus, if pure oxygen is breathed at a pressure of two atmospheres absolute, the total volume of physically dissolved oxygen in 100 ml of arterial blood is approximately 4 ml; at 3 atmospheres absolute, 6 ml, etc.

The oxygen available for cellular consumption is that dissolved in plasma. The volume of the gas normally utilized is about 6 ml per 100 ml of arterial blood, the quantity in solution at a partial pressure of 3 atmospheres absolute. At this and higher partial pressures of oxygen there is no reduction of oxyhemoglobin since the supply of dissolved gas is adequate without replenishment from that source. Under such circumstances, this function of hemoglobin has been demonstrated as unnecessary for maintenance of life.[7]

Hemoglobin normally functions in another transportational system in combining with carbon dioxide to form carbamino-hemoglobin. This process proceeds as oxyhemoglobin is reduced and is dependent upon the availability of reduced hemoglobin. When the latter remains completely saturated, this transport mechanism for carbon dioxide is impaired. The interference has been suggested[4] as a possible mechanism of oxygen toxicity, an adverse pharmacologic effect of the gas.

The concomitant use of hypothermia would favor additional solution of oxygen. Such combination of techniques has been proposed for clinical application. The added advantage of decreased metabolism provided by hypothermia would further extend the usefulness of H.O. in some situations.

The physiology of H.O. is much more extensive and complex than that presented. The various aspects of respiratory and circulatory physiology omitted in the discussion are available from standard texts. The clinically oriented monograph by Comroe and associates[8] is particularly helpful in this regard.

H.O. represents an abnormal physiologic state. The concentrations of oxygen involved impose pharmacologic effects which may oppose desired benefits. The modification of end results by the occurrence of qualitative changes associated with oxygen toxicity may necessitate the termination of H.O. in the interest of safety. This aspect of H.O. is expanded in the chapter on oxygen toxicity.

Quantitative modifications of the basic physiologic process may be occasioned by pathologic conditions imposed by disease. The existence of abnormal physiologic conditions such as limited ventilation, pulmonary edema or fibrosis and intra- or extra-pulmonary, right-to-left shunts hinder achievement of arterial tensions of oxygen quantitatively similar to those of alveolar gases. Although significant differences between the two tensions of oxygen may persist throughout H.O., the desired level of arterial oxygenation may be affected through application of higher alveolar tensions than would otherwise be necessary in the absence of the pathologic conditions. Actually, they are among those suggested as likely to be benefited by H.O. to the extent that hypoxia associated with them is relieved.

The development of elevated tensions of oxygen in arterial blood does not, per se, guarantee a proportionate rise in cellular oxygenation. Hemodynamic responses[18] affect perfusion which is a function of cardiac output and peripheral resistance. Impaired cardiac output resulting from disease, depressant drugs or the effect of oxygen itself may oppose cellular oxygenation. Debate continues regarding the vasoconstrictive potentiality of oxygen and the opposing effect of carbon dioxide. The problem is complicated by the stimulatory effect of H.O. upon the adreno-sympathetic nervous system. It is conceivable that some tissues are less well oxygenated during H.O. than presumed from known arterial tensions of the gas; some might even be rendered relatively hypoxic.

The ubiquity of the physiologic implications of H.O. is suggested from succeeding chapters, particularly that pertaining to oxygen toxicity. Its impact upon the respiratory, cardiovascular, autonomic and central nervous systems result in prominent clinical manifestations. Concomitant metabolic changes would be expected to produce generalized effects. Subtle, sub-clinical changes are presumed to precede overt manifestations.

In spite of the studies made in the development of H.O., the therapeutic regimen is still essentially experimental. Its current status is characterized by numerous, unsolved physiologic problems some of which have been the subject of investigation for many years. Most notable among these are studies of gas transport and exchange[2,4,9,13,14] and pulmonary complications[6,16,17] of H.O. Clinical observations[3,5,8,10,13,14,15,19] and animal studies [1,7,9,11] related to therapeutic applications are of increasing importance. The projection of hyperbaricity to pressures[12] greatly exceeding those now employed has begun. Succeeding chapters of the monograph provide numerous other references of physiologic significance.

Time will provide solutions for many of the pending problems. The crudeness of current instrumentation for the continuous determination of oxygen in blood and tissues is a recognized deterrent to progress. When reliable microtechniques for quantitative measurements of oxygen within cells and mitochondria become available, research will be expedited. Such instrumentation should also contribute toward more effective clinical application of H.O. and enhanced scientific evaluation of its results.

For a comprehensive and authoritative source of physiologic information, *Fundamentals of Hyperbaric Medicine* recently published by the National Research Council is recommended.

References

1. ASHMORE, P. G.: An investigation of methods of producing respiratory insufficiency in dogs in order to study the effects of treatment with high atmospheric pressure. *Med. Serv. J. Canada,* 20:500, 1964.
2. BAHNSON, H. T., AND MATTHEWS, C. M.: Blood and tissue gases of animals exposed to one and seven atmospheres of oxygen or air. *Amer. J. Physiol., 175:*87, 1953.
3. BEHNKE, A. R.: High atmospheric pressures; Physiological effects of increased and decreased pressure; Application of these findings to clinical medicine. *Ann. Intern. Med., 13:*2217, 1940.

4. BEAN, J. W.: Effect of oxygen at increased pressures. *Physiol. Rev.*, *25*:1, 1945.

5. BEHNKE, A. R., THOMSON, R. M., AND MOTLEY, E. P.: Psychologic effects of breathing air at 4 atmospheres pressure. *Amer. J. Physiol., 112*:554, 1935.

6. BENNET, G. A., AND SMITH, F. J. C.: Pulmonary hypertension in rats living under compressed air conditions. *J. Exp. Med., 59:* 181, 1934.

7. BOEREMA, I., MEIJNE, N. G., BRUMMELKAMP, W. K., BOUMA, S., MENSCH, M. H., KAMERMONS, R., HANF, S. M., AND AALDEREN, W. VANS Life without blood. *J. Cardiov. Surg., 1:*133, 1960.

8. COMROE, J. H., FORSTER, R. E., DUBOIS, A. B., BRISCOL, W. A., AND CARLSEN, E.: *The Lung.* 2nd ed. Chicago, Yr. Bk., Pub. 1962.

9. FUSON, R. L., BOINEAU, J. P., SMITH, W., SALTZMAN, H. A., SPACH, M., AND BROWN, I. W. JR.: Oxygen transport and acid-base responses of cyanotic dogs to hyperbaric oxygenation. *Clin. Res., 12*:182, 1964.

10. HERLOCHER, J. E., QUIGLEY D. G., BEHAR, V. S., SHAW, E. G., AND WELCH, B. E.: Physiologic response to increased oxygen partial pressure: I. Clinical Observations. *Aerospace Med., 35*:613, 1964.

11. LEVY, J. V., AND RICHARDS, V.: Effect of oxygen at high pressure (OHP) on asphyxial survival time of rats. *Proc. Soc. Exp. Biol. Med., 109*:941, 1962.

12. MEMBERY, J. H., AND LINK, E. A.: Hyperbaric exposure of mice to pressures of 60 to 90 atmospheres. *Science, 144*:1241, 1964.

13. LENFANT, C.: Measurement of factors impairing gas exchange in man with hyperbaric pressure. *J. Appl. Physiol., 19*:189, 1964.

14. ROBERTSON, W. G., HARGREAVES, J. J., HERLOCHER, J. E., AND WELCH, B. E.: Physiologic response to increased oxygen partial pressure. II. Respiratory studies. *Aerospace Med., 35*:618, 1964.

15. SCHAEFER, K. E.: *Environmental Effects on Consciousness.* New York, Macmillan, 1962.

16. SMITH, F. J. C., BENNETT, G. A., HEIM, J. W., THOMSON, R. M., AND DRINKER, C. K.: Morphological changes in the lungs of rats living under compressed air conditions. *J. Exp. Med., 56:*79, 1932.

17. SMITH, F. J. C., HEIM, J. W., THOMSON, R. M., AND DRINKER, C. K.: Bodily changes and development of pulmonary resistance in rats living under compressed air conditions. *J. Exp. Med., 56*:63, 1932.

18. WHALEN, R. E., SALTZMAN, H. A., HOLLOWAY, D. H., JR., MC-INTOSH, H. D., AND SIEKER, H. O.: Hemodynamic responses of hyperbaric oxygenation. *Circulation, 30: Suppl. 3:*177, 1964.

19. ZALUSKY, R., ULVEDAL, F., HERLOCHER, J. E., AND WELCH, B. E.: Physiologic response to increased oxygen partial pressure. III. Hematopoiesis. *Aerospace Med., 35:*622, 1964.

3

Oxygen Toxicity

Oxygen toxicity is a complex phenomenon which, in spite of extensive investigation over many years, remains an enigma. The possibility of adverse effects arising from the breathing of pure oxygen was first suspected by Priestley[66] in 1775, one year after his discovery of the gas. His subsequent experimentations and those of Lavoisier[56] confirmed his suspicion in their demonstrations of hemorrhagic congestions in the lungs of animals that had succumbed from prolonged inhalation of oxygen in high concentrations at atmospheric pressure. Beddoes and Watt[15] voiced their concern regarding possible dangers of its clinical application in some diseases.

It was Bert, however, who first recognized oxygen toxicity as a distinct clinical entity with adverse effects manifested by the acute onset of convulsions and death in animals subjected to inhalation of the gas at hyperbaric partial pressures. Equally important was his elucidation of the role of partial pressure in the determination of clinical events associated with the inhalation of gases and vapors. As a result of his studies, acute oxygen poisoning characterized by fatal, strychnine-like convulsions occurring within a few hours of exposure to oxygen at pressures above 3.5 atmospheres absolute became known as the "Paul Bert effect."

The subacute variety of toxicity, characterized by the development over a period of days of pulmonary damage and death associated with oxygen inhalation at lesser pressures, was termed the "Lorrain Smith effect." It was he who had reported the results of a pathological study of pulmonary effects caused by increased oxygen tensions in inspired air.

Subsequent to recognition of the clinical implications of oxygen toxicity there ensued investigative interest spurred by naval and aeronautical developments following World War I and again by the current revivification of hyperbaric therapy. There has resulted a vast literature which would justify a comprehensive critical review at this time. Such is beyond the scope of an introductory monograph. The reviews of Stadie and associates,[70] Bean,[4] and Ohlsson[64] offer excellent critiques of events up to about twenty years ago. In addition to the above, particularly noteworthy contributions have been made by Behnke,[16-21,80] Comroe,[26] Becker-Freyseng[13,14,25] and Clamann, Lambertsen,[47-54] Gerschman, [36-39,41] and their associates.

The current clinical concept of oxygen toxicity has evolved from numerous studies in human beings.[12,13,16-22,24,25,27,29,46,48-52, 54,55,61,62,80] Supportive evidence is available from animal and in-vitro investigations. Two generalizations seem justifiable: oxygen at partial pressures less than about 0.6 atmosphere is unlikely to cause toxic symptoms regardless of its percentage composition in inhaled mixtures; above approximately 0.6 atmosphere the presenting symptomatology is a function of the partial pressure and length of exposure to the gas. Continuous exposure of many hours to oxygen at partial pressures not exceeding about 2 atmospheres absolute, produces symptoms referable primarily to the respiratory system. Relatively brief exposures to the gas at partial pressures of several atmospheres or above acutely affect the central nervous system.

Comroe and his associates[27] reported substernal pain and dyspnea aggravated by exercise and coughing as the commonest symptom. The earliest onset was after four hours of continuous breathing of oxygen at atmospheric pressure; the incidence of this complaint increased in the series of normal subjects over a twenty-four-hour period. Other disorders reported were nasal congestion, otalgia, headache, joint and muscle pains, paresthesias and giddiness. No pathological pulmonary changes were detectable by radiological examination.

Investigations of H.O. by Behnke and coworkers[16-21,80] have demonstrated its acute impact upon the central nervous system. Exposures of three hours duration to oxygen at 3 atmospheres absolute were tolerated reasonably well, although progressive changes in visual acuity, a rising diastolic pressure, facial pallor and dilation of pupils were observed. Impending collapse tended to occur suddenly during the fourth hour of exposure with an abrupt rise in pulse rate, systolic and diastolic pressures, and more severe restriction of vision. Subjective feelings of dizziness, nausea and impending collapse necessitated termination of experiments.

Oxygen at 4 atmospheres absolute may cause syncope and convulsions within forty-five minutes. Behnke[17] considers the convulsive seizure as the "most striking and inexplicable event of oxygen toxicity at high pressure." An incidence of about 2 per cent has been reported in naval diving candidates exposed to oxygen at 2.8 atmospheres absolute for thirty minutes at rest. Convulsions have been reported[24] in relation to therapeutic applications of H.O.

The respiratory system has been the subject of considerable investigation in relation to H.O. The nature of pulmonary lesions[23,29,31,45,58,64,65,74,75] has been scrutinized in an effort to ascertain whether they are primarily due to the direct action of oxygen upon alveolar membranes or secondary to physiological changes in the capillary circulation. Studies[33,40,43,47-54,59,68,73,77] of the effect of H.O. upon respiratory gases in the blood and associated ionic changes are pertinent to the unsettled problem. The latter type of investigation has another significance related to a theory of oxygen toxicity first proposed by Gesell[40] and strongly favored by Bean[4,9] and Becker-Freyseng.[13] Presumably, according to the theory, the dual role of hemoglobin in transporting oxygen and carbon dioxide is adversely affected by complete saturation with oxygen, so that hypercarbia results. In support of the theory are observed elevations of the carbon dioxide contents of blood, the development of acidosis during H.O., lowering of the convulsive threshold by carbon dioxide and the protective action of alkalinization.[9,33] Contrary to the theory is the lack of convincing evidence[17,53] of development of sufficiently high levels of carbon dioxide in either blood or tissues to be responsible for observed toxic effects of H.O. A direct cellular action of oxygen is becoming increasingly suspect as its mode of toxicity.

The central nervous system[3,8,12,17,18,21,32,44,53,59,71,76] has been scrutinized because of its target role in oxygen toxicity. The same considerations of a primary toxic action upon cells versus a secondary effect of carbon dioxide apply. The vascular effects of H.O. and its effect upon circulation especially in the brain have received considerable attention not only by Lambertsen and co-

workers[47-54] but also by others.[1,44,63,67,78] Vasodilation secondary
to increased carbon dioxide content of arterial blood would favor
hyperoxygenation of cerebral tissue and a direct toxic action of
oxygen; vasoconstriction would tend to hinder excessive oxygenation. Measurements of cerebral blood flow[51-53] and studies
[18,63,67] of the visual effects of H.O. fail to indict oxygen as a
direct cause of significant vasoconstriction. The role of carbon
dioxide rather than oxygen in controlling the caliber of cerebral
vessels is stressed by Behnke.[17]

The direct effect of oxygen upon cellular activity has been
proposed as a mechanism of its toxicity. Bert[22] suggested an interference with enzymatic activity to the extent of severe metabolic
disturbance resulting from hyperoxic anoxia. Enzymatic studies
[2,28,57,70] during H.O. have indicated inhibition of some. In his
review, Stadie[70] summarized the concept of enzymatic interference as a basis of oxygen toxicity and indicated his favoring of it
in spite of admitted difficulty in reconciling the rapid onset of
convulsive activity with the relatively slow interference with enzymatic activity observed. It is conceivable that the vulnerability
of certain enzymatic processes to H.O. may eventually explain
oxygen toxicity. It may be that the time factor related to the
onset of convulsions is a function of subtle, biochemical changes
preceeding the acute clinical episode.

The release of cellular toxins has been proposed as a mechanism of action. Gerschman[36-39,41] has proposed the presence of
toxic free radicals as a cause of oxygen toxicity; observed similari-
ties of the effects of H.O. and x-irradiation have been noted.[24,38,41]

The findings of recent researches support an expanding concept of oxygen toxicity. The evidence suggests a direct, ubiquitous
[1,34,36,60] action of oxygen in the production of its toxic manifestations.

The adreno-sympathetic nervous system[5,6,10,32,37,39,42,72] seems
anatomically and physiologically related to oxygen toxicity. The
observations of Behnke and recent endocrine studies during H.O.
suggest a relationship between the onset of acute disturbance of
the central nervous system and a strong discharge of the sympathetic aspect of the autonomic nervous system. This concept is
further supported by the reported protective action of certain

drugs[6,7,35,79] antagonistic toward sympathetic activity. A sustained discharge of sympathetic hormones in lower concentrations might account for the gradual development of pulmonary complications from H.O.

The administration of oxygen to previously hypoxic persons may cause syncope. This effect, known as the "oxygen paradox" [55,62] deserves further consideration to establish its relation, if any, to oxygen toxicity.

The complexity of the phenomenon is manifested by the numerous unsolved problems related to it. Answers are likely to become available through biochemical studies of the subclinical subtleties preceeding acute clinical events. Such may be inferred from the individual presentations of C. J. Lambertsen, R. E. Forster, Niels Haugaard and J. W. Bean, and from the panel discussion of oxygen toxicity during the Symposium on Hyperbaric Oxygenation (*N.Y. Acad. Sci., 117:* Art. 2, 1965).

In the limited use of H.O. to date, a relatively small percentage of patients have convulsed. An unusual case is known which involved convulsions during H.O. and subsequently death associated with pulmonary complications suspected of having resulted from continued oxygen therapy at atmospheric pressure. Whereas the "Paul Bert" and "Lorrain Smith" effects remain distinguishable there may exist a common pharmacologic basis related to biochemic changes. Pre-clinical events leading to both types may be in progress simultaneously within the central nervous and respiratory systems. The more frequent occurrence of convulsions rather than pulmonary complications associated with H.O. is likely a matter of relative sensitivity.

Eventual understanding of subclinical biochemical events may allow their prophylactic prevention or treatment and avoidance of clinically disasterous sequelae.

References

1. ALLEN, S. C.: A comparison of the effects of nitrogen and hyperoxia on the vascular developments of the chick embryo. *Aerospace Med., 34:*897, 1963.
2. ARMSTRONG, J. M., COATES, J. H., AND MORTON, R. K.: Flavin dissociation and inactivation of cytochrome b_2 by oxygen. *Nature, 186:*1033, 1960.

3. BEAN, J. W.: Alterations in C.N.S. associated with chronic motor disabilities induced by O_2 at high pressure. *Proc. Soc. Exp. Biol. Med., 58*:20, 1945.

4. BEAN, J. W.: Effects of oxygen at high pressure. *Physiol. Rev., 25:* 1, 1945.

5. BEAN, J. W.: The hypophysis as determinant in the reaction of the mammal to oxygen at high pressure. *Amer. J. Physiol., 170*:508, 1952.

6. BEAN, J. W.: Reserpine, chlorpromazine and the hypothalamus in reaction to oxygen at high pressure. *Amer. J. Physiol., 187*:389, 1956.

7. BEAN, J. W.: Chlorpromazine, its protective action in oxygen toxicity. *Amer. J. Physiol., 198*:341, 1960.

8. BEAN, J. W.: Cerebral oxygenation with high pressure oxygen. *Amer. J. Physiol., 201*:1192, 1961.

9. BEAN, J. W.: Tris buffer, carbon dioxide, and sympathoadrenal system in reactions to high pressure oxygen. *Amer. J. Physiol., 201*:737, 1961.

10. BEAN, J. W., AND JOHNSON, P. C.: Epinephrine and neurogenic factors in the pulmonary edema and C.N.S. reactions induced by oxygen at high pressure. *Amer. J. Physiol., 180*:438, 1955.

11. BEAN, J. W., AND SIEGFRIED, E. C.: Transient and permanent aftereffects of exposure to oxygen at high pressure. *Amer. J. Physiol., 143*:656, 1945.

12. BEAN, J. W., AND WAGNER, I.: Effects of exposure to oxygen at high barometric pressure on higher functions of the C.N.S. *Proc. Soc. Exp. Biol. Med., 54*:134, 1943.

13. BECKER-FREYSENG, H.: Physiological and patho-physiological effects of increased oxygen tension: In: *German Aviation Med., World War II*. Dept. of the Air Force, pp. 493-514, 1950.

14. BECKER-FREYSENG, H., AND CLAMANN, H. G.: Zur Frage der Sauerstoffvergiftung. *Klin. Wschr., 18*:1382, 1939.

15. BEDDOES, T., AND WATT, J.: *Considerations on the Medicinal Use and on the Production of Factitious Airs*. 2nd ed., Bristol, Bulgin and Rosser, 1795.

16. BEHNKE, A. R.: High atmospheric pressures, physiological effects of increased and decreased pressure; application of these findings to clinical medicine. *Ann. Intern. Med., 13*:2217, 1940.

17. BEHNKE, A. R.: Effects of nitrogen and oxygen on consciousness. In: *Environmental Effects on Consciousness*. Ed.: K. E. Schaefer New York, Macmillan, 1962.

18. BEHNKE, A. R., FORBES, H. S., AND MOTLEY, E. P.: Circulatory and visual effects of oxygen at three atmospheres pressure. *Amer. J. Physiol., 114:*436, 1936.

19. BEHNKE, A. R., JOHNSON, F. S., POPPEN, J. R., AND MOTLEY, E. P.: Effect of oxygen on man at pressures from one to four atmospheres. *Amer. J. Physiol., 110:*565, 1935.

20. BEHNKE, A. R., SHAW, L. A. SHILLING, C. W., THOMPSON, R. M., AND MESSER, A. C.: Studies on the effects of high oxygen pressure, *Amer. J. Physiol., 107:*13, 1934.

21. BEHNKE, A. R., THOMPSON, R. M., AND MOTLEY, E. P.: The psychologic effects from breathing air at 4 atmospheres pressure. *Amer. J. Physiol., 112:*554, 1935.

22. BERT, P.: *La Pression Barometrique.* Paris, Masson, 1878. English translation by M. A. and F. A. Hitchcock, Columbus, College Book, 1943.

23. CEDERGREN, B., GYLLENSTEN, I., AND WERSÄLL, J.: Pulmonary damage caused by oxygen poisoning; An electron-microscopic study in mice. *Acta Paediat. (Upps.), 48:*477, 1959.

24. CHURCHILL-DAVIDSON, I., AND EMERY, E. W.: Investigations concerning irradiation under high pressure oxygen; Apparatus and techniques. *Proc. Roy. Soc. Med., 57:*350, 1964.

25. CLAMANN, H. G., AND BECKER-FREYSENG, H.: Einwirkung des Sauerstoffs auf den Organismus bei höherem als normalem Partialdruck unter besonderer Berücksichtigung des Menschen. *Luftfarhtmed., 4:*1, 1939.

26. COMROE, J. H., AND DRIPPS, R. D.: *The Physiological Basis for Oxygen Therapy.* Springfield, Thomas, 1950.

27. COMROE, J. H. DRIPPS, R. D., DUMKE, P. R., AND DEMING, M.: Oxygen toxicity. The effect of inhalation of high concentration of oxygen for twenty-four hours on normal men at sea level and at a simulated altitude of 18,000 feet. *J.A.M.A., 128:*710, 1945.

28. DICKENS, F.: Toxic effects of oxygen on brain metabolism and in tissue enzymes. *Biochem. J., 40:*145, 1946.

29. DOLEVAL, V.: The effect of longlasting oxygen inhalation upon respiratory parameters in man. *Physiol. Bohemoslov., 11:*149, 1962.

30. DU BOIS, A. B.: Oxygen toxicity. *Anesthesiology, 23:*473, 1962.

31. DURFEY, J. Q.: Post-mortem pulmonary changes occurring in mice exposed to 100 percent oxygen at 740 mm. Hg. *Aerospace Med., 35:*265, 1964.

32. EDSTROM, J. E., AND ROCKERT, H.: The effect of oxygen at high pressure in the histology of the central nervous system and sympathetic and endocrine cells. *Acta Physiol, Scand., 55:*255, 1962.

33. FELIG, P., AND LEE, W. L., JR.: Protective action of alkalinizing agents against oxygen toxicity in the rat. *Aerospace Med., 35:* 265, 1964.

34. FERM, V. H.: Teratogenic effects of hyperbaric oxygenation. *Proc. Soc. Exp. Biol. Med., 116:*975, 1964.

35. GARWACKI, J.: The effect of neuroplegics on the changes in respiratory organs of rats breathing pure oxygen under atmospheric pressure. *Acta Physiol. Pol., 11:*73, 1960.

36. GERSCHMAN, R., ARGUELLES, A. E., AND IBEAS, D. I.: Effects of high oxygen tensions on mammalian gonads. *Proc. Int. Union Physiol. Sci. Int., Cong., 2:*357, 1962.

37. GERSCHMAN, R. D., GILBERT, L., NYE, S. W., DWYER, P., AND FENN, W. O.: Role of adrenalectomy and adrenal-cortical hormones in oxygen poisoning. *Amer. J. Physiol., 178:*346, 1954.

38. GERSCHMAN, R. D., GILBERT, L., NYE, S. W., DWYER, P., AND FENN, W. O.: Oxygen poisoning and x-irradiation: a mechanism in common. *Science 119:*623, 1954.

39. GERSCHMAN, R., AND FENN, W. O.: Ascorbic acid content of adrenal glands of rats in oxygen poisoning. *Amer. J. Physiol., 176:*6, 1954.

40. GESELL, R.: On the chemical regulation of respiration: The regulation of respiration with special reference to the metabolism of the respiratory center and the coordination of the dual function of hemoglobin. *Amer. J. Physiol., 66:*5, 1923.

41. GILBERT, D. L., GERSCHMAN, R., AND FENN, W. O.: Effects of fasting and x-irradiation on oxygen poisoning in mice. *Amer. J. Physiol., 181:*272, 1955.

42. HALE, H. B., WILLIAMS, E. W., ANDERSON, J. E., AND ELLIS, J. P., JR.: Endocrine and metabolic effects of short-duration hyperoxia. *Aerospace Med., 35:*449, 1964.

43. HILL, L.: Influence of CO_2 in production of oxygen poisoning. *Quart. J. Exp. Physiol., 23:*49, 1933.

44. JACOBSON, I., HARPER, A. M., AND McDOWALL, D. G.: The effects of oxygen under pressure on cerebral blood-flow and cerebral venous oxygen tension. *Lancet, 2:*549, 1963.

45. JAMIESON, D., VAN DEN BRENK, H. A.: Pulmonary damage due to high pressure oxygen breathing in rats. *Aust. J. Exp. Biol. Med Sci., 40:*309, 1960.

46. KYDD, G. H., AND BETZ, L. H.: Observations on acute and chronic oxygen poisoning. *Aerospace Med., 35:273,* 1964.

47. KOUGH, R. H., LAMBERTSEN, C. J., STROUD, N. W., GOULD, R. A., AND EWING, J. H.: Some observations on the role of carbon dioxide in acute oxygen toxicity at $3\frac{1}{2}$ atmospheres inspired oxygen tension. *Amer. J. Med. Sci., 221:354,* 1951.

48. LAMBERTSON, C. J., KOUGH, R. H., COOPER, D. Y., EMMEL, G. L., LOESCHCKE, H. H., AND SCHMIDT, C. F.: Comparison of relationship of respiratory minute volume of pCO_2 and pH of blood in man during hyper-ventilation at 1 and 3 atmospheres. *J. Appl. Physiol., 5:803,* 1953.

49. LAMBERTSEN, C. J., STROUD, M. W. III, EWING, J. H., AND MACK, C.: Oxygen toxicity; effects of oxygen breathing at increased ambient pressure upon pCO_2 of subcutaneous gas depots in man, dogs, rabbits, and cats. *J. Appl. Physiol., 6:358,* 1953.

50. LAMBERTSEN, C. J.: Respiratory and circulatory actions of high oxygen pressure. Underwater physiology symposium. *National Academy of Sciences, National Research Council,* Publication *377:25,* 1955.

51. LAMBERTSEN, C. J., COOPER, D. Y., EMMEL, G. L., KOUGH, R. H., LOESCHCKE, H. H., AND SCHMIDT, C. F.: Oxygen toxicity. Effects in man of oxygen inhalation at 1 and 3.5 atmospheres upon blood gas transport, cerebral circulation and cerebral metabolism. *J. Appl. Physiol., 5:471,* 1953.

52. LAMBERTSEN, C. J. EWING, J. H., KOUGH, R. H., GOULD, R., AND STROUD, M. W. III.: Oxygen toxicity. Arterial and internal jugular blood gas composition in man during inhalation of air, 100% O_2 and 2% CO_2 at 3.5 atmospheres ambient pressure. *J. Appl. Physiol., 8:255,* 1955-56.

53. LAMBERTSEN, C. J., OWEN, S. G., WENDEL, H., STROUD, M. W., LURIE, A. A., LOCHNER, W., AND CLARK, G. F.: Respiratory and cerebral circulatory control during exercise at 0.21 and 2.0 atmospheres inspired pO_2. *J. Appl. Physiol., 14:966,* 1959.

54. LAMBERTSEN, C. J., STROUD, M. W., III, GOULD, R. A., KOUGH, R. H., EWING, J. H., AND SCHMIDT, C. F.: Oxygen toxicity. Respiratory responses of normal men to inhalation of 6 and 100 per cent oxygen and 3.5 atmospheres pressure. *J. Appl. Physiol., 5:487,* 1953.

55. LATHAM, F.: The oxygen paradox: experiments on the effect of oxygen in human anoxia. *Lancet, 1:77,* 1951.

56. Lavoisier, A. L.: *Alterations qu' eprouve láir respiré (1785)*. *Memories sur la respiration et la transpiration des animaux.* Paris, Gauthier-Villars, 1929.

57. Mann, P. J. G., and Funstel, J. H.: Toxic effects of oxygen and of hydrogen peroxide on brain metabolism. *Biochem. J., 40:*139, 1946.

58. Marcozzi, G., Messinetti, A., Colombati, M., Mocavero, G., and Zelli, G. P.: Oximetric variations and pulmonary lesions induced by inhalation of oxygen at concentrations higher than that of the atmosphere. Experimental study. *Arch. De Vecchi Anat. Pat., 32:*609, 1960.

59. Marshall, J. R., and Lambertsen, C. J.: Interactions of increased pO_2 and pCO_2 effects in producing convulsions and death in mice. *J. Appl. Physiol., 16:*1 1961.

60. Mengel, C. E., Kann, H. E., Smith, W. W., and Horton, B. D.: Effects of invivo hyperoxia on erythrocytes. Hemolysis in mice exposed to hyperbaric oxygenation. *Proc. Soc. Exp. Biol. Med., 116:*259, 1964.

61. Michel, E. L., Langevin, R. W., and Gell, C. F.: Effect of continuous human exposure to oxygen tension of 418 mm. Hg for 168 hours. *Aerospace Med., 31:*138, 1960.

62. Miles, S.: Oxygen syncope. Royal Naval Personnel Research Committee. *R.N.P., 57:*880, 1957.

63. Noell, W. K.: Effects of high and low oxygen tensions on the visual system. In: *Environmental Effects on Consciousness.* Ed. K. E. Schaefer. New York, Macmillan, 1962.

64. Ohlsson, W. T. L.: A study on oxygen toxicity at atmospheric pressure. *Acta Med. Scand.,* Suppl. *190:*1, 1947.

65. Penrod, K. E.: Nature of pulmonary damage produced by high oxygen pressures. *J. Appl. Physiol., 9:*1, 1956.

66. Priestley, J.: *Experiments* 1775.

67. Saltzman, H. A., Hart, L., Duffy, E., and Sieker, H. O.: The effects of hyperbaric oxygenation upon retinal circulation. *J.A.M.A., 188:*450, 1964.

68. Shaw, L. A., Behnke, A. R., and Messer, A. C.: Role of CO_2 in producing symptoms of oxygen poisoning. *Amer. J. Physiol., 108:*652, 1934.

69. Smith, J. L.: The pathological effects due to increase of oxygen tension in the air breathed. *J. Physiol., 24:*19, 1899.

70. Stadie, W. C., Riggs, B. C., and Haugaard, N.: Oxygen poisoning. *Amer. J. Med. Sci., 207:*84, 1944.

71. STEIN, S. N.: The neurophysiological effects of oxygen under high pressure. In: *Environmental Effects on Consciousness*. Ed. K. E. Schaefer. New York, Macmillan, 1962.

72. TAYLOR, D. W.: Effects of adrenalectomy on oxygen poisoning in the rat. *J. Physiol., 140:23,* 1958.

73. TAYLOR, H. J.: The role of CO_2 in oxygen poisoning. *J. Physiol., 109:272,* 1949.

74. TRECIOKAS, L. J.: O_2 poisoning, electron microscopy of alveolar cells. *Aerospace Med., 30:674,* 1959.

75. VAN DEN BRENK, H. A., AND JAMIESON, D.: Pulmonary damage due to high pressure oxygen breathing in rats. I. Lung weight, histologic and radiological studies. *Aust. J. Exp. Biol. Med. Sci., 40:37,* 1962.

76. VORONOV, L. B.: Brain structures and origin of convulsions caused by high oxygen pressure (HOP). *Int. J. Neuropharmacol., 3:* 279, 1964.

77. WALKER, I. G.: The involvement of carbon dioxide in the toxicity of oxygen at high pressure. *Canad. J. Biochem., 39:*1803, 1961.

78. WHALEN, R. E., SALTZMAN, H. A., HOLLOWAY, D. H., JR., McINTOSH, H. D., SIEKER, H. O., AND BROWN, I. W., JR.: Cardiovascular responses to hyperbaric oxygenation. *Clin. Res., 12:*195, 1964.

79. WOOD, J. D., AND WATSON, W. J.: Protection action of gamma-aminobutyric acid against oxygen toxicity. *Nature, 195:*296, 1962.

80. YARBROUGH, O. D., WELHAM, W., BRINTON, E. S., AND BEHNKE, A. R.: *Symptoms of Oxygen Poisoning and Limits of Tolerance at Rest and at Work.* Experimental Diving Unit, Naval Gun Factory, Washington, D. C., Project X-337, Report No. 1, 1947.

4

Decompression Sickness

THE DESIGNATION OF THIS chapter conveys an etiologic connotation of a complex disorder variously known as caisson disease, bends, chokes, divers' palsy or paralysis, itch, prickles, fits, aeropathy and compressed air illness. Hoff[18] credits Triger[23] with the report of the first cases of the disease in 1841. One of two caisson workers experienced severe pain in the left arm, and the other in the knees and left shoulder, a half hour after emerging from a pressure of 3 atmospheres absolute.

According to Amstrong,[1] Pol and Watelle[22] in 1854 reported the necessity of discharging twenty-five of sixty-four workers who could not tolerate decompression for various reasons including joint and muscle pains, cramps, vomiting, vertigo, double vision, chest pain, cough and unconsciousness. Two others died following decompression which was accomplished twice daily within one and one-half hour after periods of four hours at 4.5 atmospheres absolute. Sensing the cause to be too rapid decompression, symptoms were treated in one case by recompression.

A year later, Littleton[20] described twenty-five cases of the illness, mentioning pains in limbs and joints, paralysis and unconsciousness as manifestations of it. Recalling Robert Boyle's observation of a gas bubble in the aqueous humor of the eye of a snake that had been decompressed, he suspected the release of gas as the cause of the disease.

The list of symptoms was further extended in the review by Friedburg[11] in 1872 who mentioned pain in limbs, dyspnea, coughing, convulsions, stammering, paralysis of the legs and bladder, sudden unconsciousness and death. Convinced that the manifestations of the disease were related to the sudden release of gases dissolved during compression, he recommended slow decompression.

Except for minor cutaneous sensations of itching, prickling and formication, these early reported observations quite adequately encompass the complex symptomatology responsible for the broad nomenclature of the disease.

27

Subsequently, Bert[6] verified earlier impressions of the cause through decompression experiments with animals. The local congestion of tissues and blood with gas bubbles was confirmed. In 1900, Heller and coworkers[16] published an extensive report of the pathophysiology of decompression sickness.

Behnke and his naval associates in the 1930's were confronted with practical aspects of the disease related to diving operations. So extensive were their contributions to the literature that reference to reviews[2,3,5] containing extensive bibliographies suffices. Among their accomplishments were the elucidation of the offending role of nitrogen, practical suggestions for minimizing its effects through denitrogenation with oxygen or by its substitution with lesser soluble helium in inhaled mixtures of gases, and establishment of principles and means for treatment of the disease through recompression. As a result of their interests and experience in the treatment of decompression sickness, medical officers of naval diving units represent the foremost group of specialists in the field, whose knowledge should prove invaluable toward progress in H.O.

The past decade has witnessed a rise in the incidence of decompression sickness due to the popularity of scuba diving.[4,8,9] This fact emphasizes the increased risk of decompression associated with its application by inadequately informed personnel. Over the years, there have appeared comprehensive treatises[11,12,14,17,21] on the illness. Unfortunately, they do not meet the needs of physicians who are not specialized in the field. More appropriate to that need are several recent reports[4,8,9,19,25] which are highly recommended. As hyperbaric chambers become more available, their use in the specific treatment of victims of decompression sickness may be expected to increase. An understanding of pathophysiologic aspects of the disease[8,15,16] and its differentiation from air embolism[7] is essential to prophylaxis and rational treatment.

The basic physiologic process of decompression sickness is the local release of bubbles in tissues and blood. The principle component of the bubbles is nitrogen which during compression had been forced into solution according to the relationship between solubility and partial pressure. During faulty decompression, bubble formation as observed in the uncorking of a bottle of soda water may occur. The subject of hyperbaric treatment with oxygen is relatively protected since the latter gas is transported by hemoglobin and utilized in metabolic functions.

Symptoms do not occur in healthy persons if the pressure even after rapid decompression is not less than half that during compression.[13] Thus, relatively rapid decompression from 2 atmospheres absolute to atmospheric pressure is safe; from higher pressures decompression should be performed in stages according to details available elsewhere.[24,25]

Time is an important factor influencing risk. The maximum uptake of nitrogen by tissues is not instantaneously accomplished upon exposure to elevated pressures. Brief exposures entail less risk than prolonged ones. By the same token, repeated exposures are more dangerous than a single one during a day. This follows from the fact that complete elimination of excess nitrogen requires many hours.

Tissues have different rates of uptake of nitrogen according to their relative vascularities and rates of perfusion; the higher the perfusion rate, the faster the equilibration of tensions of the gas between tissues and alveoli.

The capacities of various tissues for dissolving nitrogen depends upon their chemical compositions. Solubility of the gas is about five times greater in lipid than in water.[8] Accordingly, nerve elements and adipose tissue have greater capacities than less fatty tissues. The rate of saturation of nervous tissue, as opposed to neutral fat deposits is favored by its greater vascularity.

Supersaturation of tissues during decompression with nitrogen probably precedes actual bubble formation. If ambient pressure is reduced to no more than half, only assymptomatic microscopic bubbles probably form. More than halving of the original pressure leads to bubble formation of symptomatic proportions. Pain, which is the commonest presenting symptom with predilection for the long bones and joints of the limbs, is considered the result of pressure within bone, periosteum and tendons.[4,8] Although this symptom usually appears within the first hour after decompression, it may be delayed to up to six hours or even longer. Muscle pains are less common.

Involvements of the central nervous system are the most serious. Considering the multiplicity of important structures and the possibility of ubiquitous bubble formation, the complexity and variability of manifestations reported are not surprising. These include paralaysis, hypalgesia, anesthesia, coma, convulsions and death. Shock resulting from neurocirculatory collapse is an accompaniment of the latter more serious consequences. Relatively, the spinal cord is more frequently involved than the brain. Residual damage may include various degrees of paralysis or anesthesia and loss of control of bladder and bowels. Such conditions are more feared than painful ones because of the anatomical sites involved. The manner of involvement of the central nervous system, whether intra- or extra-vascular, remains a subject of debate.

Although cough and a substernal burning sensation may be the extent of respiratory involvement, at times they are the precursors of the serious conditions known as the "chokes" characterized by progressive dyspnea, cyanosis, apprehension, and shock with all of its possible sequelae.

Cutaneous symptoms of itching, prickling and formication and manifestations of rash or blebs sometimes occur. The exact sites of involvements of nervous elements is speculative. A relation to subcutaneous fat deposits is suspected.

Transient blurring of vision occurring shortly after decompression is usually associated with more serious aspects of decompression sickness[8] and is considered related to vasomotor disturbances.

The issue of the relative importance of intra- versus extra-vascular bubbles in the production of symptoms and damage remains unresolved. Behnke[4] stresses the importance of intra-vascular bubbles; Dewey[8] favors an extra-vascular explanation in relation to the production of pain and central nervous system effects. The possibility of bubble embolization involving large vessels cannot be excluded in situations such as the "chokes." Such involvement of major vessels is unrelated to the phenomenon of "air embolism."[7] The latter refers to damage of overly distended lungs and the passage of air via the pulmonary veins to the left heart and thence via the carotid arteries to the brain.

Prophylaxis against decompression sickness is preferable to treatment which may not always affect a complete cure. Prophylaxis involves appropriate decompression procedure patterned upon a regimen such as that advised in the *U.S. Navy Diving Manual*[24] but modified according to the needs of personnel of lesser physical fitness than healthy young sailors.

The uniquely effective treatment of decompression sickness is appropriate recompression and gradual decompression. Oxygen inhalation during decompression favors nitrogen elimination. It should be helpful during delay from the time of onset of symptoms to that of recompression, but should not be the limit of treatment of the disease. Delays in recompression mitigate its effectiveness and increase the possibility of permanent damage. The disease constitutes a medical emergency and should be treated as such.

Candidates for hyperbaric participation require screening through thorough physical examinations including radiological evidences of the conditions of sinuses and joints of the long bones. Those with respiratory or cardiovascular diseases are advisedly excluded. Periodic radiological examinations of bones, especially those about the knees may reveal evidence of subclinical bone disease in those subjected to repeated decompressions. Such precautionary measures have legal as well as medical connotations.

Because of its lesser solubility than nitrogen, helium has been employed in deep sea diving.[10] The use of large chambers for H.O. would seem to preclude the use of the gas by personnel concerned with the care of patients. The use of masks for its administration would impose serious interferences, especially for surgical teams. The cost of charging the chambers and replenishing the atmosphere with the gas would impose technical and economic impracticalities. The use of oxygen for the same purpose would be attended with the prohibitive dangers of toxicity and fire. Under the circumstances, the best recourse is employment of established rules for decompression with the operation controlled by persons thoroughly trained in their execution.

In this age of private ownership of planes, the urge to fly in an unpressurized craft soon after a decompression might conceivably lead to symptoms of decompression sickness which might have been averted at ground level. This is because tissues with sluggish circulation are relatively slow in discharging the gases stored during compression. The precaution applies to scuba divers as well as those concerned with hyperbaric therapy.

Pulmonary barotrauma resulting in pneumathorax is a serious consequence of inappropriate decompression. Congenital cysts, scar tissue vesicles, pulmonary emphysema and bronchitis are considered predisposing causes. Behnke[4] cited an occurrence in a trainee who "blew-up" on submarine escape. Loss of consciousness, stertorous, gasping respiration, bloody frothing from the mouth, dilated pupils and fixed, deviated eyes characterized the event. Life was saved through prompt recognition of the etiology, recompression and removal of 2,250 ml of air from the left side of the thorax during recompression before reduction to atmospheric pressure.

Yanda[26] emphasized the possibility of pulmonary barotrauma occurring in emphysematous persons and warns of the danger associated with exposures of elderly persons to compression — decompression procedures. In an outline of the management of moderately severe to far advanced emphysema, he included the use of bronchodilator drugs preceding decompression, intermittent aerosol administration of such drugs during decompression, consistent monitoring of the patients' pulmonary status and a maximal, minute-by-minute rate of decompression of 0.5 psi.

The seriousness of decompression sickness behooves the reporting by all members of the team of untoward symptoms and intensification of observations of the patient. Such is particularly desirable in cases of suspected impairment of pulmonary function in the latter. Decompression rates are necessarily limited by the level of greatest intolerance among all concerned.

References

1. ARMSTRONG, H. G.: Principles and Practice of Aviation Medicine. 3rd ed. Baltimore, Williams & Wilkins, 1952.
2. BEHNKE, A. R.: Investigations concerned with problems of high altitude flying and deep diving: Applications of certain findings pertaining to physical fitness to the general military service. *Milit. Surg., 90*:9, 1942.

3. BEHNKE, A. R.: Decompression sickness. *Milit. Med., 117*:257, 1955.

4. BEHNKE, A. R.: Problems in the treatment of decompression sickness (and traumatic air embolism). *Ann. N.Y. Acad. Sci., 117*: 843, 1965.

5. BEHNKE, A. R., AND STEPHENSON, C. S.: Applied physiology. *Ann. Rev. Physiol., 4*:575, 1942.

6. BERT, P.: *La Pression Barometrique.* Paris, Masson, 1878. English translation by M. A. and F. A. Hitchcock, Columbus, College Book Co., 1943.

7. COLLINS, J. J., JR.: An unusual case of air embolism precipitated by decompression. *New Eng. J. Med., 266*:595, 1962.

8. DEWEY, A. W. JR.: Decompression sickness, an emerging recreational hazard. *New Eng. J. Med.,* Part I, *267*:759, 1962. Part II, *267*:812, 1962.

9. DUFFNER, G. J.: Scuba diving injuries: Predisposing causes and prevention. *J.A.M.A., 175*:375, 1961.

10. END, E.: The use of new equipment and helium gas in a world record dive. *J. Ind. Hyg., 20*:511, 1938.

11. FRIEDBERG, H.: Ueber die Rücksicten der öffentlichen Gesundheitzpflege auf das Arbeiten in comprimirter Luft. *Dinglers J., 205*: 509, 1872.

12. FULTON, J. F. (ed.) : *Decompression Sickness. Caisson Sickness, Diver's and Flier's Bends and Related Syndromes.* Philadelphia, Saunders, 1951.

13. HALDANE, J. S.: *Respiration.* New Haven, Yale, 1922.

14. HAYMAKER, W.: Decompression sickness. In: *Scholz' Handbuch der Speziellen Pathologischen Anatomie und Histologie.* Munich, Springer, Vol. *14*, (Text in English), 1955.

15. HAYMAKER, W., AND JOHNSON, A. D.: Pathology of decompression sickness. *Milit. Med., 117*:285, 1955.

16. HELLER, R., MAGER, W., AND VON SCHRÖTTER, H.: *Luftdruckerkrankungen: mit Besonderer Berücksichtigung der Sogenannten.* (2 vol). Vien, Alfred Hölder, 1900.

17. HILL, L.: *Caisson Sickness.* London, Arnold, 1912.

18. HOFF, E. C.: *A bibliographical Source-Book of Compressed Air, Diving and Submarine Medicine.* ONR, U.S. Gov't. Printing Office, 1948.

19. LANPHIER, E. H.: Diving medicine. *New Eng. J. Med., 256*:120, 1957.

20. LITTLETON, T.: Effects of submarine descent. *Ass. Med. J., 3*:127, 1855.

21. NATIONAL RESEARCH COUNCIL: *Decompression Sickness.* Philadelphia, Saunders, 1951.

22. POL, B., AND WATELLE, T. J.: Mémoire sur les effects de la compression de l'air appliquée au creusement des puits á houille. *Ann. Hyg. Publ. Paris,* Series 2, *1*:241, 1854.

23. TRIGER, E.: Memoire sur un appareil á air comprimé, pour le percement des puits de mines et autres travous, sous les laux et dans les sobles submergés. *C.R. Acad. Sci. (Paris), 13*:884, 1841.

24. *U.S. Navy Diving Manual (Part 1):* U. S. Navy Dept., Washington, D.C., U.S. Gov't. Printing Office, 1959.

25. WORKMAN, R. D.: Standard decompression procedures and their modification in preventing the bends. *Ann. N.Y. Acad. Sci., 117*:834, 1965.

26. YANDA, R. L.: Comment in panel discussion. *Ann. N.Y. Acad. Sci., 117*:713, 1965.

5

Nitrogen Narcosis

Nitrogen under pressure is capable of depressing the central nervous system. Damant,[8] in 1930, and Hill and Phillips,[10] in 1932, observed personality changes and impairment of mental and motor functions in individuals subjected to the breathing of air under hyperbaric conditions. Although the effects have been characterized as a slowing of cerebration, at pressures approaching 10 atmospheres absolute loss of consciousness has occurred.

More appropriate to the circumstances of modern H.O. were the observations of Behnke[2,3] and associates derived from a study conducted at 4 atmospheres absolute. Even under these conditions, there occurred changes in mood frequently manifested as euphoria, fixation of ideas, evidences of stupefaction, and difficulties in recollection and concentration. Manual dexterity also was impaired. Characteristically, the time of onset of these effects was only a few minutes after exposure to hyperbaric inhalation of air.

Shilling and Willgrube[15] applied psychological tests to determine the effects of compressed air upon the sensorium. At 4 atmospheres absolute there were increases in time and errors associated with solution of arithmetic problems. Both tended to increase with further progressions of pressure.

Bennett and Glass[5,6] reported electroencephalographic changes after compression to 4 atmospheres absolute. Their studies indicated an abolition of blocking of alpha rhythm and depression of flicker fusion frequency. Again, these effects already evident at 4 atmospheres absolute, increased with further elevations of pressure.

The incrimination of nitrogen as the gas responsible for the observed depression of psychological and motor functions required differentiation of its potentialities in this respect from those of oxygen and carbon dioxide.

The exclusion of oxygen was relatively simple. In air compressed at 4 atmospheres absolute, the partial pressure of oxygen would be only 0.8 of an atmosphere. Barely within the probable range of toxicity, the onset of symptoms would not be expected for hours. Symptoms of oxygen toxicity referable to the respiratory rather than the central nervous system would be expected. Furthermore, the substitution of helium[2,4,9] for nitrogen in mixtures with oxygen inhaled under pressure eliminated depressant effects observed under similar conditions of breathing compressed air. Likewise, the abolition of blocking of alpha rhythm in electroencephalograms does not occur if helium is substituted for nitrogen in the inspired air. These evidences excluded oxygen as the offending gas and strongly suggested the action of nitrogen. There remained proof of the narcotic potentiality of nitrogen and the exclusion of carbon dioxide as the causative agent.

The narcotic potentiality of nitrogen is implicated in the complex problem concerning the mechanism of action of anesthetics. Behnke and his associates[3] considered it in accord with the Meyer-Overton theory which relates narcotic potencies of drugs with their relative partition coefficients between oil and water. Carpenter,[7] in his studies of the effects of "inert" gases under pressure, has provided convincing evidences of the potentiality of hyperbaric nitrogen. The supportive evidences provided by recent studies of xenon anesthesia have been cited.[2,12] Particularly convincing is the profound degree of anesthesia possible with xenon under hyperbaric conditions[13] at 3 atmospheres absolute. The lesser, though significant, depressant effect attributed to nitrogen at 4 atmospheres absolute is understandable.

Narcosis subsequent to increased arterial tensions of carbon dioxide associated with the breathing of compressed air has been postulated.[1] The unimportance of the gas in this respect has been convincingly presented.[14,16] The opposing evidence is based upon the relatively minor elevations of tensions of carbon dioxide and persistence of narcotic effects when tensions of the gas return toward normal during continued breathing of compressed air.

Pressures of 4 atmospheres absolute have been employed during surgical procedures. The use of even higher pressures may be contemplated.

Inherent dangers of nitrogen narcosis reside not only in the nature of its effects but also in the speed of their onset. Effects are apparent within a few minutes after exposure to hyperbaric air. Two factors are responsible for the speedy events. The body is already saturated with nitrogen at a partial pressure of about 0.8 atmosphere. Beginning with this high level of saturation, elevations of the tension of the gas proceed directly with increases in pressure. The uptake is accumulative with no substitution of gases involved. Secondly, the low solubility of nitrogen favors the rapid onset of narcotic effects in accordance with the theoretical considerations of Kety.[11]

The implications of the rapid onset of nitrogen narcosis is that there is little time after reaching appropriate pressures for the performance of tasks uninfluenced by it.

Nitrogen narcosis has been likened to intoxication from alcoholic beverages. Divers have related sensations at various depths with numbers of martinis consumed on other occasions. The problem is complicated by the impaired judgment of those affected who might be unaware of it or deny their incompetencies under the circumstances. Assurances of capabilities offered by persons narcotized by nitrogen would offer no guarantee of ability in performance.

The implications of the psychological impact of nitrogen narcosis in H.O. are obvious. From available evidence, the possibility of minimal effects cannot be excluded at 4 atmospheres absolute. Different individuals would tend to vary in their responses. The performance of a particular person cannot be judged, a priori, from previous performances of others. Neither would the same response be expected of a person on different exposures to the same pressure.

The problem is a serious one especially if higher pressures than now employed are anticipated for the future. The impracticalities associated with the substitution of nitrogen in air with oxygen or helium have been presented previously. Direction of activities within a chamber and assurance of their proper execution from the exterior would be difficult. Some such supervision might, however, be profitably attempted. Perhaps at least one member of a team within a chamber could be accommodated with a mask to breathe a helium-oxygen or other non-noxious mixture of gases, if pressures are employed which would impose serious hazards from nitrogen narcosis.

References

1. BEAN, W. J.: Tensional changes of alveolar gas in reactions to rapid compression and decompression and question of nitrogen narcosis. *Amer. J. Physiol., 161:*417, 1950.

2. BEHNKE, A. R.: Effects of nitrogen and oxygen on consciousness. In: *Environmental Effects on Consciousness.* New York, Macmillan, 1962.

3. BEHNKE, A. R., THOMPSON, R. M., AND MOTLEY, E. P.: The psychologic effects from breathing air at four atmospheres pressure. *Amer. J. Physiol., 112:*554, 1935.

4. BEHNKE, A. R., AND YARBROUGH, O. D.: Physiologic studies of helium. *U.S. Nav. Med. Bull., 36:*542, 1938.

5. BENNETT, P. B.: Flicker fusion frequency and nitrogen narcosis. A comparison with EEG changes and the narcotic effects of nitrogen mixtures. Admiralty Report R.N.P.L., 5, 1958.

6. BENNETT, P. B., AND GLASS, A.: The electroencephalograph and narcosis under high partial pressure of nitrogen and isonarcotic concentrations of nitrous oxide. Admiralty Report R.N.P.L., *11:*57, 1957.

7. CARPENTER, F. G.: Anesthetic action of inert and unreactive gases on intact animals and isolated tissues. *Amer. J. Physiol., 178:* 505, 1954.

8. DAMANT, G. C. C.: Physiological effects of work in compressed air. *Nature, 126:*606, 1930.

9. END, E.: The use of new equipment and helium gas in a world record dive. *J. Ind. Hyg., 20:*511, 1938.

10. HILL, L., AND PHILLIPS, A. E.: Deep sea diving. *J. Roy. Nav. Med. Serv., 18:*165, 1932.

11. KETY, S. S.: The theory and applications of the exchange of inert gas of the lungs and tissues. *Pharmacol. Rev., 3:*1, 1951.

12. LAWRENCE, J. H., LOOMIS, W. F., TOBIAS, C. A., AND TURPIN, F. H.: Preliminary observations on the narcotic effect of xenon with review of values for solubilities of gases in water and oils. *J. Physiol., 105:*197, 1946.

13. PITTINGER, C. B., FAULCONER, A. JR., KNOTT, J. R., PENDER, J. W., MORRIS, L. E., AND BICKFORD, R. G.: Electroencephalographic and other observations in monkeys during xenon anesthesia at elevated pressures. *Anesthesiology, 16:*551, 1955.

14. RASHBASS, C.: The unimportance of carbon dioxide in nitrogen narcosis. Admiralty Report R.N.P.L., 11, 1955.
15. SHILLING, C. W., AND WILLGRUBE, W. W.: Quantitative study of mental and neuromuscular reactions as influenced by increased air pressure. *U.S. Nav. Med. Bull., 35:*373, 1937.
16. TAYLOR, H. J.: Neurophysiological effects of nitrogen. In: *Environmental Effects on Consciousness.* New York, Macmillan, 1962.

6

Clinical Applications: Status of the Literature

THE FIRST CLINICAL APPLICATION of H.O. in recent times was reported by Churchill-Davidson and his associates[6] a decade ago in relation to the radiotherapy of tumors. Soon thereafter, there appeared the report by Boerema and his associates[4] pertaining to oxygen drenching as an adjunct to cardiac surgery. It was not, however, until 1961 that the medical profession became widely interested. The occasion was the simultaneous publication in Surgery of two papers: the one by Boerema[2] concerned his hyperbaric operating chamber; the other by Brummelkamp[5] related to the treatment of anaerobic infections. The following year the press introduced the public to H.O., thus further extending and intensifying interest in it. Subsequently there seems to have been an exponential expansion in the volume of literature.

Several publications are particularly worthy of noting. Among the various reviews, that pertaining to H.O. and current medical uses of oxygen by Barach[1] is authoritatively outstanding. The first volume of specific clinical orientation appeared in 1964 under the editorship of Boerema aand associates.[3] It is a compilation of the Proceedings of the First International Congress on H.O. held in Amsterdam during September, 1963. Numerous original and review articles by prominent clinical investigators are presented.

Equally impressive and broader in scope was the important conference sponsored jointly by the New York Academy of Sciences and the National Academy of Sciences in February, 1964. The preceedings of the conference, which contained much of clinical significance, have recently been published by the New York Academy of Sciences.[8]

Another innovation is the Hyperbaric Medicine Newsletter which has been launched on a bimonthly basis by the State University of New York at Buffalo, School of Medicine. The stated intention is to provide news items pertaining to hyperbaric medicine on an international scope.

The recent publication, *Fundamentals of Hyperbaric Medicine*,[7] should be of value to all users of hyperbaric equipment.

A perusal of the literature is quite revealing in a number of respects. Firstly, whereas the sources of information are expanding, most clinical applications of H.O. are still the accomplishments of original investigators in the respective fields. Secondly, there is considerable duplication of material published by authors in different journals. Thirdly, an appreciable quantity of information is of a contemplative nature, presumably assembled in anticipation of eventual research or clinical application. Fourthly, a large portion pertains to preliminary animal experimentation. Fifthly, the actual numbers of areas of clinical application and the sizes of most series relevant to each are still quite limited. Sixthly, the creditable attitude of responsible researchers is one of caution based upon the conviction that clinical developments to date remain in the experimental stage. Seventhly, apparent results in the various areas of application vary widely; some evoke enthusiasm; others warrant continued clinical research; in at least one, abandonment of the technique seems likely. Eighthly, generally there is need for controlled data to allow valid comparisons of results with those obtained by conventional therapy.

Subsequent chapters dealing with specific clinical applications have been provided with sufficiently comprehensive bibliographies to allow pursuit in detail of the summarizations presented. Purposely omitted are references to many anonymous articles and editorials which seem to pervade both medical and secular publications. In each instance an attempt has been made to provide an understanding of the rationale serving as the working hypothesis in clinical development.

References

1. BARACH, A. L.: Hyperbaric oxygen and current medical uses of oxygen. *New York J. Med., 63:*2775, 1963.
2. BOEREMA, I.: An operating room with high atmospheric pressure *Surgery, 49:*291, 1961.
3. BOEREMA, I., BRUMMELKAMP, W. H., AND MEIJNE, N. G., (eds.) : *Clinical Application of Hyperbaric Oxygen.* Proceedings of the First International Congress, Amsterdam, Sept., 1963. New York, Elsevier, 1964.

4. BOEREMA, I., KROLL, J. A., MEIJNE, N. G., LOKIN, E., KROON, B., AND HUISKES, J. W.: High atmospheric pressure as an aid to cardiac surgery. *Arch. Chir. Neerl., 8:*193, 1956.
5. BRUMMELKAMP, W. H.: Treatment of anaerobic infections in pressure chamber. *Surgery, 49:*299, 1961.
6. CHURCHILL-DAVIDSON, I., SANGER, C., AND THOMLINSON, R. H.: High pressure oxygen and radiotherapy. *Lancet, 1:*1091, 1955.
7. *Fundamentals of Hyperbaric Medicine.* Washington, D. C., National Research Council, 1965.
8. Hyperbaric Oxygenation. *Ann. N.Y. Acad. Sci., 117:*Art. 2, 1965.

7

Cancer Therapy

CONSIDERING THE IMPORTANCE of this field of medicine, it is not surprising that early attention had been given to the application of H.O. Credit for development of the rationale upon which such application has been based is due to Gray and his associates.[14-16] According to their theorization, confirmed by laboratory experimentation, the radiosensitivity of a normal cell rendered hypoxic declines to about one third of its original level. On the other hand, hyperoxygenation of a normal cell produces only a relatively small increase in sensitivity.

Assuming the presence within a tumor of a small percentage of hypoxic cells which during conventional radiotherapy might escape destruction and subsequently resume mitosis, Churchill-Davidson and his associates[6] first applied H.O. during irradiation. The inhalation of oxygen during radiotherapy to bolster its effect was not new; administration of the gas at hyperbaric pressures was an innovation. The results in the several cases of terminal, massive cancer were gratifying in the degree of resolution of those parts of the tumor irradiated during H.O. as compared with portions treated at ordinary tensions of oxygen. Subsequently, their studies were extended[3-5,7,10-12,21,24] with modifications in technique, and continued basic research.

Initially, patients were anesthetized prior to their confinement in a metal chamber with limited ports for viewing. The development of transparent chambers has led to increased treatment of premedicated but unanesthetized patients. Oxygen at 3 atmospheres absolute seems favored.[3] Higher pressures have been employed, especially in anesthetized persons in whom convulsions as a manifestation of oxygen toxicity are considered less likely to occur. Convulsions without serious consequences have been reported.

H.O. is not considered a panacea in the radiotherapy of all tumors. Those of squamous cell origin have been particularly responsive. Impressive regressions have been noted in malignancies inolving the neck, pharyngeal structures and associated nodes. Excessive pulmonary fibrosis has resulted after irradiation of bronchogenic carcinoma during H. O.

Certain basic scientific and clinical information is essential for valid comparisons of the benefits of H.O. in radiotherapy with results achieved by conventional therapy. There is need for development of reliable techniques for measuring oxygen tensions within tumors in order to ascertain the degree of oxygenation produced by H.O. Cater and his associates[1,2] are pursuing this important matter. Their animal researches have demonstrated the fallacy of assuming significant elevation of tensions in all tissues subsequent to exposure to H.O.

Sedatives, anesthetics and hyperbaric oxygen itself are known to produce variable cardiovascular effects. Until their influences upon perfusion are known, there can be no assurance of optimal oxygenation of tissues presumed from known tensions of the gas in arterial blood. Correctable physical factors such as positioning and temperature might benefit perfusion and improve clinical results.

The results of efforts in this initial area of clinical application of H.O. warrant continued study. While impressions are gratifying, the benefits of H.O. in radiotherapy lack comparison with results of conventional therapy. Controlled data are lacking for want of paired tumors of the types investigated. Larger series of cases from broader sources[8,13,18,20,22,23,25,26] of clinical investigation combined with follow-up data of recurrences will eventually afford comparative information.

Chemotherapy of cancer is becoming increasingly important among investigations aimed toward combating the disease. The possible benefits of combined H.O. and chemotherapy are being investigated.[9,17,19] The incipient phases of these laboratory studies preclude statements of their possible clinical value.

Although the increase in irradiation sensitivity of normal tissue is presumed to be small with H.O., determinations of its consequences are indicated. Concannon[8] has reported significant renal effects which deserve consideration in therapy. Adverse effects of H.O. upon other organs exposed to radiotherapy are not known.

References

1. CATER, D. B., SCHOENIGER, E. L., AND WATKINSON, D. A.: Effect on oxygen tensions of tumors of breathing oxygen at high pressures. *Lancet, 2:*381, 1962.
2. CATER, D. B., AND SILVER, I. A.: Quantitative measurements of oxygen tension in normal tissues and in the tumors of patients before and after radiotherapy. *Acta Radiologica (Stockholm), 53:*233, 1960.
3. CHURCHILL-DAVIDSON, I.: The small patient chamber, radiotherapy. *Ann. N.Y. Acad. Sci., 117:*875, 1965.
4. CHURCHILL-DAVIDSON, I., AND EMERY, E. W.: Investigations concerning irradiation under high pressure oxygen: Apparatus and techniques. *Proc. Roy. Soc. Med., 57:*350, 1964.
5. CHURCHILL-DAVIDSON, I., FOSTER, C. A., AND THOMLINSON, R. H.: High-pressure oxygen and radiotherapy. *Med. World (London), 88:* (2) :125, 1958.
6. CHURCHILL-DAVIDSON, I., SANGER, C., AND THOMLINSON, R. H.: High pressure oxygen and radiotherapy. *Lancet, 1:*1091, 1955.
7. CHURCHILL-DAVIDSON, I., SANGER, C., AND THOMLINSON, R. H.: Oxygenation in radiotherapy: Clinical application. *Brit. J. Radiol., 30:*406, 1957.
8. CONCANNON, J. P., SUMMERS, R. E., BREWER, R., WEIL, C., AND HAYESLIP, D.: High oxygen tension and radiation effect on the kidney. *Radiology, 82:*508, 1964.
9. DeCOSSE, J. J., AND ROGERS, L. S.: Effect of hyperbaric oxygen and cancer chemotherapy on growth of animal tumors. *Surg. Forum, 15:*203, 1964.
10. EMERY, E. W.: Irradiation of conscious patients under high pressure oxygen. *Lancet, 1:*248, 1960.
11. EMERY, E. W., AND LUCAS, B. G. B.: Instrumental and technical notes: The irradiation of conscious patients under high pressure oxygen. *Brit. J. Radiol., 37:*475, 1964.
12. EMERY, E. W., LUCAS, B. G. B., AND WILLIAMS, K. G.: Technique of irradiation of conscious patients under increased oxygen pressures. *Lancet, 1:*248, 1960.
13. GOLDFEDER, A., AND CLARKE, G. E.: The response of neoplasm to x-irradiation in vivo at increased oxygen tension. *Radiat. Res., 13:*751, 1960.
14. GRAY, L. H.: Oxygenation in radiotherapy. Radiobiological considerations. *Brit. J. Radiol., 30:*403, 1957.

15. GRAY, L. H.: Radiobiologic basis of oxygen as a modifying factor in radiation therapy. *Amer. J. Roentgen., 85:*803, 1961.

16. GRAY, L. H., CONGER, A. D., EBERT, M., HORNSEY, S., AND SCOTT, O. C. A.: The concentration of oxygen dissolved in tissues at the time of irradiation as a factor in radiotherapy. *Brit. J. Radiol., 26:*638, 1953.

17. KINSEY, D. L.: Hyperbaric oxygen and 5-fluorouracil in the treatment of experimental melanoma. *Surg. Forum, 15:*205, 1964.

18. MALLAMS, J. T., BALLA, G. A., FINNEY, J. W., AND ARONOFF, B. L.: Regional oxygenation and irradiation, head and neck. *Arch. Otolaryng. (Chicago), 79:*155, 1964.

19. NATHANSON, L., BROWN, B., MADDOCK, C., AND HALL, T.: Effects of anti-tumor agents at hyperbaric oxygen in normal and tumor bearing rodents. *Clin. Res., 12:*465, 1964.

20. POWERS, W. E., AND TOLMACH, L. J.: Demonstration of an anoxic component in a mouse tumor-cell population by in vivo assay of survival following irradiation. *Radiology, 83:*328, 1964.

21. SANGER, C.: High pressure oxygen and radiation therapy. *Amer. J. Roentgenol., 81:*498, 1959.

22. SEEMAN, W. B.: Combined high pressure O_2 and radiation in cancer. *Amer. J. Roentgen., 85:*816, 1961.

23. SEEMAN, W. B., TAPLEY, N. DU V., SANGER, C., JACOX, H. W., AND ATKINS, H. L.: Combined high-pressure oxygen and radiation therapy in the treatment of human cancer. *Amer. J. Roentgen., 85:*816, 1961.

24. THOMLINSON, R. H.: An experimental method for comparing treatments of intact malignant tumors in animals and its application to the use of oxygen in radiotherapy. *Brit. J. Cancer, 14:*555, 1960.

25. VAN DEN BRENK, H. A. S.: Effect of high pressure oxygen on radiosensitivity of Ehrlich's tumor in mice after "Immunological Approximation." *Brit. J. Cancer, 15:*61, 1961.

26. WILDERMUTH, O.: Hybaroxic radiation therapy in cancer management. *Radiology, 82:*767, 1964.

8

Surgery

Tɪᴍᴇ ɪs ᴀ ʟɪᴍɪᴛɪɴɢ ғᴀᴄᴛᴏʀ poignantly related to certain cardiovascular and neuro-surgical procedures involving temporary occlusion of circulation in vital organs. Extension of this limiting factor by hyperoxygenation of tissues prior to occlusion of circulation has been the outstanding contribution of H.O. to surgery. Coupled with hypothermia, which favors oxygen solubility and simultaneously reduces metabolic requirements of the gas, its benefits may be augmented.

Pioneering investigations of the surgical potentialities of H.O. were initiated by Boerema and his associates[10] in Amsterdam. Their subsequent researches[8-12,19,20] and clinical applications indicate their continued leadership in the field. In pre-clinical animal studies, they demonstrated the feasibility of extending the safe temporal limits of arterial occlusion, the possibility of briefly sustaining life without blood, the benefits of H.O. combined with extracorporeal circulation and/or hypothermia, and the value of H.O. in the prophylaxis and treatment of fibrillation during hypothermia. Cautious clinical application of H.O. followed and has continually expanded. Particularly in the definitive correction of cardiovascular defects in infants and children has H.O. yielded gratifying results. Their accomplishments in the use of the technique as an adjunct to the surgical management of gas gangrene are accounted in the chapter devoted to anaerobic and other infections. A pressure of 3 atmospheres absolute has been generally employed by these investigators.

Interest in surgical applications of H.O. was next evident in reports from Glasgow where Illingworth, Smith and their associates[15,21,24-26] began early laboratory investigations leading to clinical usage. This group of investigators has had a particular interest in the preservation of cerebral cortical activity during vascular occlusion. In addition to their applications of H.O. in the correction of congenital cardiac defects, they have been favorably impressed by results obtained in the management of peripheral injuries involving extensive vascular impairment. In the latter situations, it was felt that less extensive surgery was required due to the preservation of tissue by the adjunctive use of H.O.

In the United States, Bernhard and his coworkers at Boston [1-6,27] have likewise employed H.O. with encouraging results in the correction of congenital cardiac lesions. Similar application has been made by Brown[13] at Durham where he and Smith[14] have given extensive consideration to safety features in the design and operation of hyperbaric chambers. Their recommendations and admonitions deserve consultation by anyone concerned in hyperbaric research or clinical application. Other groups[7,16-18, 22,23] are involved in preparatory phases of research of surgical implication.

Organ transplantation currently provokes a high degree of surgical interest. Among the major problems involved are preservation of organs from the moment of removal to the time of transplantation, and immunologic factors affecting their rejection by the host. With regard to preservation, some early studies[7,17,18] suggest possible benefits of H.O. combined with hypothermia. The eventual role of H.O. in this aspect of transplantation surgery will depend upon the nature of the balance between the destructive and preservative properties of oxygen upon enzymatic activity. A prolongation of physiologic integrity would stimulate the development of organ banks and allow elective rather than emergency scheduling of transplantation procedures, thus extending their availability.

Consideration has been given to the possible combination of H.O., extracorporeal circulation and hypothermia. Except in rare instances involving prolonged occlusion of cerebral circulation, it is difficult to conceive needs for such combination in clinical practice. Oxygen toxicity might be a limiting factor.

From the above presentation, it is evident that the benefits of H.O. to surgery are restricted to a relatively few indications, principally the correction of congenital cardiac defects. Its importance in this respect is subject to changes. Development of satisfactory pump oxygenators specifically designed for infant use would probably result in their replacement of H.O. in cardiac surgery. Contrariwise, interest in the application of H.O. in the preserva-

tion of organs preceeding transplantation and in transplantation
procedures themselves will probably increase. If its potentialities
in this regard prove to be substantial, the status of H.O. as an
adjunct to surgery will be significantly enhanced.

References

1. BERNHARD, W. F.: Current status of hyperbaric oxygenation in
   pediatric surgery. *Surg. Clin. N. Amer., 44:*1583, 1964.
2. BERNHARD, W. F.: Hybaroxic surgery; An adjunct in the management of congenital cardiovascular disease. *Dis. Chest, 46:*114,
   1964.
3. BERNHARD, W. F., FRITTELLI, G., TANK, E. S., AND CARR, J. G.:
   Surgery under hyperbaric oxygenation in infants with congenital cardiac disease. *Circulation, 29:*91 (Suppl.), 1964.
4. BERNHARD, W. F., AND TANK, E. S.: Effect of oxygen inhalation at
   3.0 to 3.6 atmospheres absolute upon infants with cyanotic
   congenital heart disease. *Surgery, 54:*203, 1963.
5. BERNHARD, W. F., TANK, E. S., FRITTELLI, G., AND GROSS, R. E.:
   Experimental and clinical cardiovascular surgery under hyperbaric conditions. *Proc. New Eng. Cardiov. Soc., 21:*31, 1962-63.
6. BERNHARD, W. F., TANK, E. S., FRITTELLI, G., AND GROSS, R. E.:
   The feasibility of hypothermic perfusion under hyperbaric
   conditions in the surgical management of infants with cyanotic
   congenital heart disease. *J. Thorac. Cardiov. Surg., 46:*651,
   1963.
7. BLOCH, J. H., MANAX, W. G., EYAL, Z., AND LILLEHEI, R. C.: Heart
   preservation in vitro with hyperbaric oxygenation and hypothermia. *J. Thorac. Cardiov. Surg., 48:*969, 1964.
8. BOEREMA, I.: An operating room with high atmospheric pressure.
   *Surgery, 49:*291, 1961.
9. BOEREMA, I.: Observation during operation on deeply cyanotic
   young children breathing oxygen at 3 atmospheres absolute.
   *Pediat. Surg., 52:*796, 1962.
10. BOEREMA, I., KROLL, J. A., MEIJNE, N. G., LOKIN, E., KROON, B.,
    AND HUISKES, J. W.: High atmospheric pressure as an aid to
    cardiac surgery. *Arch. Chir. Neerl., 8:*193, 1956.
11. BOEREMA, I., MEIJNE, N. G., BRUMMELKAMP, W. K., BOWMA, S.,
    MENSCH, M. H., KAMERMANS, R., STERN, H. M., AND AALDEREN,
    W. VAN.: Life without blood - a study of the influence of
    atmospheric pressure and hypothermia on dilution of the
    blood. *J. Cardiov. Surg., 1:*133, 1960.

12. BOEREMA, I., MEIJNE, N. G., AND VERMEULEN-CRANCH, D. M. E.:
    Observations during operations on deeply cyanotic young
    children breathing oxygen at 3 atmospheres absolute. *Surgery,*
    *52:*796, 1962.
13. BROWN, I. W.: Oxygen therapy at superatmospheric pressure.
    *J.A.M.A., 183:*397, 1963.
14. BROWN, I. W., AND SMITH, W. W.: General safety features in
    chamber design and operation. *Ann. N.Y. Acad. Sci., 117:*801,
    1965.
15. ILLINGWORTH, C. F. W., SMITH, G., LAWSON, D. D., LEDINGHAM, I.
    McA., SHARP, G. R., GRIFFITHS, J. C., AND HENDERSON, C. I.:
    Surgical and physiological observations in an experimental
    pressure chamber. *Brit. J. Surg., 49:*222, 1961.
16. JACOBSON, I., BLOOR, K., McDOWALL, D. G., AND NORMAN, J. N.:
    Internal carotid endarterectomy at 2 atmospheres of pressure
    *Lancet, 2:*546, 1963.
17. LILLEHEI, R. C., *et. al.*: In vitro preservation of whole organs by
    hypothermia and hyperbaric oxygenation. *Cryobiology, 1:*181,
    1964.
18. MANAX, W. G., BLOCH, J. H., LONGERBEAM, J. K., AND LILLEHEI,
    R. C.: Successful 24 hour in-vitro preservation of canine kid-
    neys by the combined use of hyperbaric oxygenation and hypo-
    thermia. *Surgery, 56:*275, 1964.
19. MEIJNE, N. G., SLUYTER, M. E., AND BOEREMA, I.: Spontaneous
    defibrillation during deep hypothermia under high atmos-
    pheric pressure. *Arch. Chir. Neerl., 14:*131, 1962.
20. MEIJNE, N. G., VERMEULEN-CRANCH, D. M. E., SLUYTER, M. E.,
    ELOFF, S. J. P., SCHRIPSEMA, L., DEEN, L., SCHOEMAKER, G., AND
    BOEREMA, I.: Experimental cardiac surgery under high atmos-
    pheric pressures. *J. Thorac. Cardiov. Surg., 44:*749, 1962.
21. PINKERTON, H. H.: The scope of a pressure chamber in surgery
    and anaesthesia. *Canad. Anaesth. Soc. J., 9:*389, 1962.
22. RICHARDS, V., PINTO, D., AND COOMBS, P.: Considerations and uses
    of hyperbaric oxygen therapy in surgery. *Amer. J. Surg., 106:*
    114, 1963.
23. RICHARDS, V., PINTO, D., AND COOMBS, P.: Studies in suspended
    animation by hypothermia combined with hyperbaric oxygen-
    ation. *Ann. Surg., 158:*349, 1963.
24. SMITH, G., LAWSON, D. D., RENFREW, S., LEDINGHAM, I. McA., AND
    SHARP, G. R.: Preservation of cerebral cortical activity by
    breathing oxygen at 2 atmospheres of pressure during cerebral
    ischemia surgery. *Surg. Gynec. Obstet., 113:*13, 1961.

25. SMITH, G., LEDINGHAM, I. McA., NORMAN, J. N., DOUGLAS, T. A., BATES, E. H., AND LEE, F. D.: Prolongation of the time of "safe" circulatory arrest by preliminary hyperbaric oxygenation and body cooling. *Surg. Gynec. Obstet., 117:*411, 1963.

26. SMITH, G., STEVENS, J., GRIFFITHS, J. S., AND LEDINGHAM, I. McA.: Near avulsion of foot treated by replacement and subsequent prolonged exposure of patient to oxygen at 2 atmospheres pressure. *Lancet, 2:*1122, 1961.

27. SMITH, R. M., CROCKER, D., AND ADAMS, J.: Anesthetic management of patients during surgery under hyperbaric oxygenation. *Anesth. Analg., 43:*766, 1964.

9

Anaerobic and Other Infections

IT IS CONSISTENT WITH REASON to suspect that organisms such as
clostridium welchii and clostridium tetani, which thrive under
conditions of low oxygen tension, might be adversely affected by
hyperoxygenation. The hypothesis is not of recent origin. According to Brummelkamp,[7] as early as 1938 oxygen had been inject-
ed into healthy tissue surrounding areas infected with gas gangrene in order to halt the advance of the disease. In 1941, De
Almeida and Pacheco studied the effect of H.O. on experimental
gas gangrene; the results of the study were not encouraging.

The first report[2] of Boerema and Brummelkamp in 1960
initiated a series of subsequent ones[1,3,4,6-13] concerning their
laboratory investigations and clinical accomplishments in the applications of H.O. in the treatment of gas gangrene. Their results
have been very impressive. In a series of thirty-seven cases[7] involving eight deaths, demise was directly due to the disease in one
instance, and probably so in two others; in the five other cases
morbid conditions prevailed from other causes.

Considering the vascular impairment prevalent in each case
of gas gangrene, the stated objective of Brummelkamp has been to
achieve the highest pressure presumed to be safe. Accordingly,
three exposures of two hours duration at three atmospheres absolute on the first day, and two similar sessions on each of the
next two days has proved to be a satisfactory regimen. Anti-gas
gangrene serum is not generally employed. Antibiotics (penicillin and/or streptomycin) are considered advisable to counteract
concurrent infections. Surgery is preferably delayed until after
the hyperbaric treatments. Marked systemic improvement is not
uncommon after the first treatment, and cure is believed to be
affected within the first day.

Encouraged by the reports from Amsterdam, other medical
centers[5,22,28,29,33-35] have undertaken treatment of gas gangrene
with H.O., in some instances using different time - pressure rela-
tionships.

The results of treatment of clostridium welchii infections with H.O. have been so encouraging that the technique promises to revolutionize the therapy of gas gangrene.

The press release[14] in 1962 concerning the hyperbaric treatment of lockjaw crisis provoked considerable medical[15] and lay attention. Based upon knowledge[37] of the oxygen lability of tetanolysin, clinical investigation of the value of H.O. in the treatment of tetanus was initiated by Pascale and his associates. [32,34] In their series of nine cases, they reported elimination of seizures, regression of symptoms and arrest of the disease. Improvement was reported after the first treatment of two hours duration at 2 to 3 atmospheres absolute. Treatments were repeated upon return of symptoms. Although most of the patients had received T.A.T., penicillin and various sedatives, the authors suggest that the antitoxin probably isn't necessary.

Winkel and Kroon[36] in their series of seven cases were likewise favorably impressed with results obtained and concluded that H.O. seems very logical in the treatment of tetanus. Repeated treatments of one and one-half hours at 3 atmospheres absolute were employed, repeated several times daily if necessary.

Brummelkamp[6] in his report of seven cases of tetanus was impressed with the beneficial effect of H.O. in the relief of trismus, but felt that the natural course of the disease was not so strikingly altered as in clostridium welchii infections.

Although the available evidence is not conflicting, neither is it satisfactorily convincing. The total number of treated cases of tetanus is small; in most, the therapeutic effect of H.O. is masked by conventional therapy. The suggestive evidence certainly seems to warrant continued research. Even though it may not be totally curative, its adjunctive use may prove to be of considerable value toward decreasing the persistent high mortality rate associated with the disease.

Little is known of the possible effects of H.O. upon other organisms, or their toxins, responsible for illnesses. Laboratory investigations of this nature are in progress. Common pathogenic bacteria,[20,21,26,30] fungi,[20,27] viruses,[24,25,31] Mycobacterium tuberculosis[17,19] and Mycobacterium leprae[17] are current targets of research. Some inhibition of growth of coagulase-positive and coagulase-negative strains of staphyloccoci, escherichia coli, candida albicans, aspergillus fumigatus and proteus bacilli have been reported. The incipient phases of these investigations, however, preclude predictions of the probable value of H.O. in combating diseases caused by the organisms.

The very broad field of infectious diseases offers numerous opportunities for research of the effect of H.O. upon them. In-vitro and animal studies are logical, initial phases of investigation. Even in the treatment of anaerobic infections, continued basic research seems desirable and would likely be profitable. Whereas the hyperbaric treatment of gas gangrene has yielded very fine results, much more seems desirable in the case of tetanus.

References

1. BOEREMA, I., AND BRUMMELKAMP, W. H.: Breathing of pure oxygen under pressure in the treatment of anaerobic infections. *Nederl. T. Geneesk., 104:*2548, 1960. Abstracted in *J.A.M.A., 175:*219, 1961.

2. BOEREMA, I., AND BRUMMELKAMP, W. H.: Treatment of anaerobic infections by inhalation of oxygen under a pressure of 3 atmospheres. *Nederl. T. Geneesk., 104:*2548, 1960.

3. BOEREMA, I., AND BRUMMELKAMP, W. H.: Inhalation of oxygen at 2 atmospheres for clostridium welchii infections. *Lancet, 2:* 990, 1962.

4. BOEREMA, I., AND BRUMMELKAMP, W. H.: Treatment of anaerobic infections by inhalation of oxygen under extremely high pressure. *Presse Med., 69:*439, 1961.

5. BRAKEBUSCH, C. O.: Gas gangrene; A case report. *Med. Bull. U.S. Army Europe, 21:*113, 1964.

6. BRUMMELKAMP, W. H.: Hyperbaric oxygen therapy in tetanus. In: *Clinical Application of Hyperbaric Oxygen.* Ed: Boerema, *et al.* New York, American Elsevier, 1964. p 63.

7. BRUMMELKAMP, W. H.: Treatment of infections with clostridium welchii by oxygen therapy at 3 atmospheres - a report on 37 cases. Ibid., p 20.

8. BRUMMELKAMP, W. H.: Treatment of anaerobic infections in pressure chamber. *Surgery, 49:*299, 1961.

9. BRUMMELKAMP, W. H.: The importance of administration of oxygen under atmospheric positive pressure in the treatment of gas phelgmon. *Nederl. T. Geneesk., 105:*2430, 1961.

10. BRUMMELKAMP, W. H.: Anaerobic infections. *Bull. Int. Chir., 21:* 481, 1962.
11. BRUMMELKAMP, W. H., HOGENDIJK, J., AND BOEREMA, I.: Treatment of anaerobic infections (clostridial myositis) by drenching the tissues with oxygen under high atmospheric pressure. *Surgery, 49:*299, 1961.
12. BRUMMELKAMP, W. H., BOEREMA, I., AND HOGENDIJK, J.: Treatment of clostridial infections with hyperbaric oxygen drenching. *Lancet, 1:*235, 1963.
13. BRUMMELKAMP, W. H., AND HEINS, H. F.: Een acute vorm van voortschrijdend huidgangreen (type meleney) en haar conservatieve behandeling door middel van doordrenking van de weefsels met zuurstof met behulp van een hyperpressie-tank. *Nederl. T. Verlosk., 63:*246, 1963.
14. EDITORIAL: For lockjaw crisis: high pressure oxygen. *Time, 79:*58, 1962.
15. EDITORIAL: Tank treatment for tetanus "sensationalized" by press. *J.A.M.A., 181:*35, 1962.
16. FREDETTE, V.: Action de l'oxygene hyperbare sur le bacille tetanique et sur la toxine tetanique. *Rev. Canad. Biol., 23:*241, 1964.
17. GOTTLEIB, S. F.: The possible use of high pressure oxygen for the treatment of leprosy and tuberculosis. *Dis. Chest, 44:*215, 1963.
18. GOTTLEIB, S. F., ROSE, N. R., MAURIZI, J., AND LANPHIER, E. H.: Hyperbaric oxygen effects on the tubercle bacillus. *Dis Chest, 46:*114, 1964.
19. GOTTLEIB, S. F., ROSE, N. R., MAURIZI, J., AND LANPHIER, E. H.: Oxygen inhibition of growth of mycobacterium tuberculosis. *J. Bact., 87:*833, 1964.
20. GOTTLEIB, S. F., ROSE, N. R., MAURIZI, J., AND LANPHIER, E. H.: Inhibitory effects of hyperbaric oxygen on bacteria and fungi. ..*Lancet, 1:*382, 1964.
21. HOPKINSON, W. I., AND TOWERS, A. G.: Effects of hyperbaric oxygen on some common pathogenic bacteria. *Lancet, 2:*1361, 1963.
22. ILLINGWORTH, C.: The Lister lecture, 1964: Wound sepsis-from carbolic acid to hyperbaric oxygen. *Canad. Med. Ass. J., 91:* 1041, 1964.
23. JACOBSEN, D. S., AND SCHWARTZ, S. I.: Effect of hyperbaric oxygenation on hepatic inflow occlusion. *Surg. Forum, 15:*198, 1964.
24. KOMANDENKO, N. I.: Effect of oxygen under pressure on the course

of experimental tick-borne encephalitis in white mice. *Vop. Virus.,* 658, 1962.

25. LIBET, B., AND SIEGEL, B. V.: Response of a virus-induced leukemia in mice to high oxygen tension. *Cancer. Res., 22:*6, 1962.

26. MCALLISTER, T. A., STARK, J. M., NORMAN, J. N., AND ROSS, R. M.: Inhibitory effects of hyperbaric oxygen on bacteria and fungi. *Lancet, 2:*1040, 1963.

27. MCALLISTER, T. A., STARK, J. M., NORMAN, J. N., AND ROSS, R. M.: Inhibitory effects of hyperbaric oxygen on bacteria and fungi. *Lancet, 1:*499, 1964.

28. MOON, A. J., WILLIAMS, K. G., AND HOPKINSON, W. I.: Infective gangrene surrounding an empyema wound treated with hyperbaric oxygen. *Brit. J. Dis. Chest, 58:*198, 1964.

29. NUCKOLLS, J. G., AND OSTERHOUT, S.: The effect of hyperbaric oxygen on anaerobic bacteria. *Clin. Res., 12:*244, 1964.

30. OLLODART, R. M., AND BLAIR, E.: The rationale for hyperbaric oxygen in the management of sepsis. *J.A.M.A., 188:*450, 1964.

31. PANOV, A. G., AND REMEZOV, P. I.: The effect of oxygen under pressure on the course of various experimental neurovirus infections in white mice. *Pop. Virusel, 5:*267, 1960.

32. PASCALE, L., WALLYN, R. J., GOLDFEIN, S., AND GUMBINER, S. H.: Treatment of tetanus by hyperbaric oxygenation. *J.A.M.A., 189:*408, 1964.

33. SMITH, G., SILLAR, W., NORMAN, J. N., LEDINGHAM, I. McA., BATES, E. H., AND SCOTT, O. C. A.: Inhalation of oxygen at 2 atmospheres for clostridium welchii infections. *Lancet, 2:*756, 1962.

34. WALLYN, R. J., GUMBINER, S. H., GOLDFEIN, S., AND PASCALE, L. R.: The treatment of anaerobic infections with hyperbaric oxygen. *Surg. Clin. N. Amer., 44:*107, 1964.

35. WEALE, F. E.: Inhalation of oxygen at 2 atmospheres for clostridium welchii infections. *Lancet, 2:*887, 1962.

36. WINKEL, C. A., AND KROON, T. A. J.: Experiences with hyperbaric oxygen treatment in tetanus. In: *Clinical Application of Hyperbaric Oxygen.* Ed.: Boerema, *et al.* New York, Elsevier, 1964. p 52.

37. WRIGHT, G. P.: Neurotoxins of clostridium botulinum and clostridium tetani. *Pharmacol. Rev., 7:*413, 1955.

10

Resuscitation; Poisonings; Asphyxia Neonatorum; Cardiac Arrest

RESUSCITATION REFERS TO REVITALIZATION of the apparently dead or the revival of depressed physiologic functions such as respiration, circulation and consciousness. Resuscitative efforts, though frequently rewarding in the saving of life, leave much to be desired. The rationale for the use of H.O. is the restoration of adequate oxygenation to hypoxic tissues. The successes achieved by conventional methods of oxygen therapy suggested the possibilities of speedier and more efficient means toward the end through hyperbaric techniques. The potentialities of H.O. have been considered in the treatment of carbon monoxide, cyanide and barbiturate poinsonings, asphyxia neonatorum and cardiac arrest.

Carbon monoxide is a lethal gas perenially responsible for a considerable number of accidental and suicidal deaths. Its toxicological action is competition on an equi-molecular basis with oxygen for combination with hemoglobin. The much greater stability of carboxyhemoglobin than oxyhemglobin accounts for the high degree of toxicity of the gas. In addition, the presence of carboxyhemoglobin causes a shift to the left of the oxygen dissociation curve. The competitive relationship between carbon monoxide and oxygen was elucidated by Haldane[14] in 1895. Subsequently, on the basis of experimental studies[11,26] the use of H.O. was suggested as a method of treatment.

The first such clinical application in acute carbon monoxide poisoning was that of Smith and Sharp[35] in 1960. Encouraging successes resulted from previous experimental work[23] at Glasgow where active research and clinical application have continued. [9,10,22,24,33,34,36] Their criteria for use of H.O. in carbon monoxide poisoning are unconsciousness or respiratory and/or circulatory depression. Oxygen is administered through a mask with a non-rebreathing valve at 2 atmospheres absolute until carboxyhemoglobin is no longer detectable in blood by which time consciousness has usually returned. Blood clearance time varies from about twenty minutes to three hours. Clearance time seems related to time of exposure to carbon monoxide rather than the blood level of carboxyhemoglobin or clinical condition of patients. Rate of clearance with H.O. at 2 atmospheres absolute is almost twice that achieved by conventional treatment with carbogen.[9,10,]

The results of treatment of carbon monoxide poisoning with H.O. have been so encouraging as to warrant the construction of a mobile hyperbaric unit to allow initiation of treatment enroute to the hospital.

Subsequent to the reported success at Glasgow, interest spread to Amsterdam.[29-30] Clinical results were considered excellent following mild poisoning but less impressive after severe intoxication. Oxygen at 3 atmospheres absolute was used, though 2 atmospheres absolute is now advocated.[30]

The classical treatment of Chen and Rose[4] for cyanide poisoning utilizes a nitrite to convert hemoglobin to methemoglobin, so that the latter may combine with cyanide ions to form cyanmethemaglobin, a complex of relatively low toxicity. Sodium thiosulfate is also advocated to allow conversion of cyanide to thiocyanate, likewise to lower toxicity. In view of the decrease in hemoglobin, H.O. would tend to support oxygenation of tissues through the increased amount of dissolved gas.

Levine[25] and Cope[5] reported evidence of the benefit of oxygen at atmospheric pressure in the treatment of laboratory animals poisoned with cyanide. Ivanov[19] has utilized H.O. at 2.8 atmospheres absolute in laboratory studies of cyanide poisoning with significant success. Although no clinical applications of H.O. in the treatment of acute cyanide poisoning are known, its use would seem rational and likely beneficial when combined with the nitrite-thiosulfate regimen.

Barbiturate poisoning is associated with tissue hypoxia resulting from depression of the respiratory and circulatory systems. Illingworth and his associates[18,27] have demonstrated marked clinical improvement of rapid onset following the initiation of H.O. at 2 atmospheres absolute in cases of severe barbiturate intoxication. Their observations suggest an expansion of the use of H.O. for this purpose.

Effective resuscitation of the newborn demands adequate oxygenation without undue delay. Impressed by delays, inadequacies, and dangers associated with routine methods of artificial ventilation, with or without intubation, and of difficulties associated with training personnel in its proper execution, Hutchison[15,16,17] conceived the use of the hyperbaric chamber as a means for accomplishing adequate oxygenation. From experimental studies of rats rendered apneic with thiopental sodium, H.O. was found effective in improving the cardiovascular status even though the animals were not actively ventilated. It has long been known that the molecular activity of gases allow their diffusion into the patent respiratory system and subsequent perfusion into the blood stream.

In a series of cases treated by placing depressed infants in a chamber compressed with oxygen at 2 atmospheres absolute, impressive results were reported by Hutchison in the initiation of respiration and rapid clinical improvement. In his experience, the longest exposure of H.O. required was thirty-four minutes. Success was reported[15] even in situations where infants were apneic in spite of suction, oxygen by face mask and analeptics. The technique is employed if after four minutes, spontaneous respiration has not begun. The limited exposure of short duration, until adequate spontaneous respiration begins, has not led to decompression problems. For the same reason, the development of retrolental fibroplasia or other manifestations of oxygen toxicity are considered unlikely. The hyperbaric technique of infant resuscitation has aroused interest in others,[1,2,6,7,8,13] especially in England. Barrie[2] has objected to the lack of arterial oxygen determinations considered essential for an accurate evaluation of the benefits of H.O. Goodlin[12] has reported some success in promoting respiration in apneic fetal mice after their immersion in an oxygen-pressurized salt solution wherein cutaneous respiration is presumed to occur. Whether or not the technique will prove superior to conventional treatment remains to be determined.

Proof is required that H.O. affords more prompt and better

tissue oxygenation and lesser residual atelectasis than occurs in expertly managed resuscitative efforts by conventional methods.

Resuscitation of patients who have suffered cardiac arrest is a most challenging problem. Hypoxia subsequent to cessation of circulation demands rapid rectification if irreparable damage is to be avoided. The rationale for treatment is the probability of achieving more rapid and effective tissue oxygenation with an elevated partial pressure of oxygen than would be likely under routine methods of oxygen administration. Koch and Vermeulen-Cranch[21] report the treatment of such a case with success. The benefits of H.O., however, were masked by other treatments including urea for reduction of cerebral edema. The seriousness of refractive cases deserves additional consideration of the possible benefits of H.O. alone and in conjunction with hypothermia as adjunctive therapy.

References

1. ALLAN, D.: Recent advances in pediatric inhalation therapy. *Surg. Clin. N. Amer., 44*:1611, 1964.

2. BARRIE, H.: Hyperbaric oxygen in resuscitation of the newborn. *Lancet, 2*:1223, 1963.

3. BROOM, B.: Hyperbaric oxygenation in resuscitation. *Lancet, 1*: 830, 1964.

4. CHEN, K. K., AND ROSE, C. L.: Treatment of acute cyanide poisoning. *J.A.M.A., 162*:1154, 1956.

5. COPE, C.: The importance of oxygen in the treatment of cyanide poisoning. *J.A.M.A., 175*:1061, 1961.

6. DAVIS, J. A., AND TIZARD, J. P. M.: Hyperbaric oxygen in resuscitation of the newborn. *Lancet, 1*:166, 1964.

7. DAWES, G. S., AND CROSS, K. W.: Hyperbaric oxygen in resuscitation of the newborn. *Lancet, 2*:910, 1964.

8. DONALD, I.: Hyperbaric oxygen in resuscitation of the newborn. *Lancet, 2*:1383, 1963.

9. DOUGLAS, T. A., LAWSON, D. D., LEDINGHAM, I. McA., NORMAN, J. N., SHARP, G. R., AND SMITH, G.: Carbon-monoxide poisoning; A comparison between the efficiences of oxygen at 1 atmosphere pressure, of oxygen at 2 atmospheres pressure and of 5% and 7% carbon dioxide in oxygen. *Lancet, 1*:68, 1962.

10. DOUGLAS, T. A., LAWSON, D. D., LEDINGHAM, I. McA., NORMAN, J. N., SHARP, G. R., AND SMITH, G.: Carbon monoxide poison-

ing. In: *Clinical Application of Hyperbaric Oxygen*. Ed., Boerema *et al*. New York, Elsevier, 1964.

11. END, E., AND LONG, C. W.: Oxygen under pressure in carbon monoxide poison. *J. Industr. Hyg. Toxicol., 24:*302, 1942.

12. GOODLIN, R. C.: Cutaneous respiration in a newborn-resuscitator: Preliminary report. *Minnesota Med., 46:*1227, 1963.

13. GOODLIN, R. C., AND PERRY, D.: Hyperbaric oxygen in resuscitation of asphyxiated newborn rabbits. *Lancet, 2:*1124, 1964.

14. HALDANE, J. S.: The relation of the action of carbonic oxide to oxygen tension. *J. Physiol., 18:*201, 1895.

15. HUTCHISON, J. H., AND KERR, M. M.: Treatment of asphyxia neonatorum by hyperbaric oxygenation. *Ann. N.Y. Acad. Sci., 117:* 706, 1965.

16. HUTCHISON, J. H., KERR, M. M., WILLIAMS, K. G., AND HOPKINSON, W. I.: Hyperbaric oxygen in the resuscitation of the newborn. *Lancet, 2:*1019, 1963.

17. HUTCHISON, J. H., KERR, M. M., WILLIAMS, K. G., AND HOPKINSON, W. I.: Hyperbaric oxygen in resuscitation of the newborn. *Lancet, 1:*225, 1964.

18. ILLINGWORTH, C. F. W., SMITH, G., LAWSON, D. D., LEDINGHAM, I. McA., SHARP, G. R., GRIFFITHS, J. C., AND HENDERSON, C. I.: Surgical and physiological observations in an experimental pressure chamber. *Brit. J. Surg., 49:*222, 1961.

19. IVANOV, K. P.: Effect of elevated oxygen pressure on animals poisoned with potassium cyanide. *Farmakol. Toksik., 22:*476, 1959.

20. JACOBINZER, H.: Carbon monoxide poisoning. *New York J. Med., 62:*2714, 1962.

21. KOCH, A., AND VERMEULEN-CRANCH, D. M. E.: The use of hyperbaric oxygen following cardiac arrest. *Brit. J. Anaesth., 34:* 738, 1962.

22. LAWSON, D. D.: Treatment of experimental CO poisoning in pressure chamber. *Lancet, 1:*800, 1961.

23. LAWSON, D. D., McALLISTER, R. A., AND SMITH, G.: The effect of high pressure oxygen in experimental acute carbon monoxide poisoning. *Scot. Med. J., 4:*327, 1959.

24. LAWSON, D. D., McALLISTER, R. A., AND SMITH, G.: Treatment of acute experimental carbon-monoxide poisoning with oxygen under pressure. *Lancet, 1:*800, 1961.

25. LEVINE, S.: Oxygen in the therapy of cyanide poisoning. *J.A.M.A., 170:*1585, 1959.

26. PACE, N., STRAJMAN, E., AND WALKER, E. L.: Acceleration of carbon monoxide elimination in man in high pressure oxygen. *Science, 111:*652, 1950.

27. PINKERTON, H. H.: The scope of a pressure chamber in surgery and anaesthesia. *Canad. Anaesth. Soc. J., 9:*389, 1962.

28. SELIGMAN, S. A.: Hazards facing the neonate. *Proc. Roy. Soc. Med., 56:*1019, 1963.

29. SLUYTER, M. E., AND BOEREMA, I.: The treatment of carbon monoxide poisoning by administration of oxygen under pressure. *Nederl T. Geneesk., 106:*826, 1962.

30. SLUYTER, M. E.: The treatment of carbon monoxide poisoning by administration of oxygen at high atmospheric pressure. *Proc. Roy. Soc. Med., 56:*1002, 1963.

31. SLUYTER, M. E.: Carbon monoxide poisoning. In: *Clinical Application of Hyperbaric Oxygen.* Proceedings of the First International Congress, Amsterdam, Sept., 1963. New York, Elsevier 1964. p 166.

32. SMITH, G.: Treatment of CO poisoning in pressure chamber. *Lancet, 2:*905, 1960.

33. SMITH, G.: Carbon monoxide poisoning. *Ann. N.Y. Acad. Sci., 117:*684, 1965.

34. SMITH, G., LEDINGHAM, I. McA., SHARP, G. R., NORMAN, J. N., AND BATES, E. H.: Treatment of coal-gas poisoning with oxygen at 2 atmospheres pressure. *Lancet, 1:*816, 1962.

35. SMITH, G., AND SHARP, G. R.: Treatment of carbon-monoxide poisoning with oxygen under pressure. *Lancet, I* 905, 1960.

36. SMITH, G., SHARP, G. R., AND LEDINGHAM, I. McA.: Treatment of coal-gas poisoning in humans by oxygen under pressure. *Scot. Med. J., 6:*339, 1961.

11

Cardiovascular Insufficiency

THE HIGH INCIDENCE OF occurrence and mortality of myocardial infarction are compelling reasons for investigating the potentialities of H.O. in the treatment of the ischemic insult. The objective of its application is amelioration of the hypoxic myocardium during development of collateral circulation. Problems inherent in hyperbaric therapy relate to means for administering oxygen continuously and avoidance of its toxicity.

A tremendous interest has been manifested in the experimental production of acute coronary occlusion in dogs and its treatment with H.O. Smith and his associates[4,11,17,23-24] and Meijne and coworkers[18-21] have been outstanding investigators in this field of experimental work. Similar interests have more recently become widespread.[5-10,13,14,16,22,25-27]

It should be stressed that the various animal studies have been concerned primarily with the effects of H.O. administered for several hours after infarction. Pressures from 2 to 4 atmospheres have been employed. Among the observations of the various investigators except Hunter and coworkers,[10] there is general agreement that H.O. decreases mortality significantly; the incidence and severity of arrhythmias is reduced; blood pressure and cardiac output are better maintained. Trapp and Creighton[25,26] and Petropoulus[21] have produced evidence suggesting a reduction in the size of the infarction in dogs treated with H.O. Harris and Hitchcock[7] have found the integrity of the SGOT test maintained during hyperbaric treatment.

The impressive results reported from animal experiments have not been realized in relatively limited clinical applications. The largest controlled series has been reported by Cameron and associates.[4] Oxygen at 2 atmospheres absolute was continuously administered for forty-eight hours to eighteen cases of acute myocardial infarction. Results were compared with eighteen controls. Overall mortality in both groups during the first six weeks after infarction were similar in that one third of each group died.

Half of the deaths in each group likewise died during the first forty-eight hours. Deterioration of two patients in the hyper-oxygenated group occurred rapidly during decompression. The mortality figures were similar to those in patients treated in the same medical unit by conventional methods during the previous 10 years. No harmful effects from H.O. were observed.

In spite of the above disappointing results in the clinical treatment of myocardial infarction with H.O., the benefits observed in experimental situations will undoubtedly prompt further trials. Alterations in technique and length of administration of H.O. may yield more encouraging clinical results.

The benefits of H.O. in the treatment of pulmonary disease[8] and especially pulmonary embolism[2,15] are being investigated. On the basis of meager evidence to date, additional investigation is encouraged.

Results of treatment of arteriosclerotic ischemia with H.O. at 2 atmospheres absolute for several hours daily over a period of two to three weeks have been disappointing, according to Illingworth, although relief of pain was achieved in some patients suffering from chronic obliterative vascular disorders.[11,12] He has been favorably impressed by results obtained in the treatment of traumatic ischemia.

Hopefully, in all aspects of cardiovascular disease, results derived from continued research will be more fruitful than the limited clinical applications to date have been.

References

1. Agustsson, M. H., Baffes, T. G., Ketola, F. H., and Baffes, C. G.: Effect of hyperbaric oxygenation on shunts, hypoxia, and cyanosis. *Circulation, 30:*39, Suppl. 3, 1964.
2. Attar, S. M. A., *et al.*: Hyperbaric oxygenation in massive pulmonary embolism. *Surg. Forum, 15:*200, 1964.
3. Boerema, I., Brummelkamp, W. H., and Meijne, N. G.: *Clinical Application of Hyperbaric Oxygen.* Proceedings of the First International Congress, Amsterdam, Sept., 1963. New York, Elsevier, 1964.
4. Cameron, A. J. V., Gibb, B. H., Ledingham, I. McA., McGuinness, J. B., Norman, J. N., and Sharif, M.: A controlled clinical trial of hyperbaric oxygen in the treatment of acute myocardial infarction: Preliminary results. Ref. 3 above, p. 75.

5. GAGE, A.: Discussion. Ref. 3 above, p. 122.
6. GAGE, A. A., FEDERICO, A. J., LANPHIER, E. H., AND CHARDACK, W. M.: Reduction by hyperbaric oxygenation of the mortality from ventricular fibrillation following experimental coronary artery ligation. *Circulation, 30:*80, Suppl 3, 1964.
7. HARRIS, R. H., AND HITCHCOCK, C. R.: Serum transaminase (SGOT) in dogs with induced myocardial infarction treated with hyperbaric oxygenation. Ref. 3 above, p. 110.
8. HITCHCOCK, C. R., HARRIS, R. H., AND HAGLIN, J. J.: Hyperbaric oxygenation in cardiac and pulmonary disease. *Dis. Chest, 44:* 622, 1963.
9. HOLLOWAY, D. H., JR., WHALEN, R. E., McINTOSH, H. D., SALTZMAN, H. A., AND BROWN, I. W., JR.: Hyperbaric oxygenation in the treatment of acute myocardial infarction in dogs. *Clin. Res., 12:*185, 1964.
10. HUNTER, S. W., LONG, S. V., AND BERGER, E. C.: Coronary occlusion, total and subtotal, under normal and hyperbaric conditions. Ref. 3 above, p. 105.
11. ILLINGWORTH, C.: Treatment of arterial occlusion under oxygen at two atmospheres pressure. *Brit. Med. J., 2:*1271, 1962.
12. ILLINGWORTH, C.: Arterial insufficiency and hyperbaric oxygenation. *Ann. N.Y. Acad. Sci., 117:*671, 1965.
13. JACOBSON, J. H., II, *et al.*: Hyperbaric oxygenation: Diffuse myocardial (sic) infarction. *Arch. Surg., 89:*905, 1964.
14. JACOBSON, J. H.: Discussion. Ref. 3 above, p. 121.
15. JUST-VIERA, J. O., AND YEAGER, G. H.: Massive pulmonary embolism. IV. The value of hyperbaric oxygen as therapy. *J. Thorac. Cardiov. Surg., 48:*185, 1964.
16. KUHN, L. A., KLINE, H., YAMAKI, T., WANG, M., AND JACOBSON, J. H.: Hemodynamic and metabolic effects of hyperbaric oxygenation in acute myocardial infarction. *Circulation, 30:*108, Suppl. 3, 1964.
17. LEDINGHAM, I. McA.: Some clinical and experimental applications of high pressure oxygen. *Proc. Roy. Soc. Med., 56:*999, 1963.
18. MEIJNE, N. G., BULTERIJS, A., ELOFF, S. J. P., AND BOEREMA, I.: An experimental investigation into the influence of administration of oxygen under increased atmospheric pressure upon coronary infarction. *J. Cardiov. Surg., 4:*521, 1963.
19. MEIJNE, N. G., BULTERIJS, A. B., SCHOEMAKER, G., AND ELOFF, S. J. P.: Treatment of dogs with oxygen under high atmospheric pressure after ligation of the descending branch of the left coronary artery. *Dis. Chest, 44:*234, 1963.

20. MEIJNE, N. G., SCHOEMAKER, G., AND BULTERIJS, A. B.: Oxygen supply to ischemic myocardial tissue under increased atmospheric pressure. Ref. 3 above, p. 69.

21. PETROPOULUS, P. C.: Influence of hyperbaric oxygenation on the haemodynamic changes and mortality after circumflex coronary artery occlusion. Ref. 3 above, p. 84.

22. ROSHE, J., AND ALLEN, W.: Effects of hyperbaric oxygenation on left circumflex coronary artery occlusion in dogs. *Surg. Forum, 15:*208, 1964.

23. SMITH, G., AND LAWSON, D. D.: Experimental coronary arterial occlusion; effects of the administration of oxygen under pressure. *Scot. Med. J., 3:*346, 1958.

24. SMITH, G., AND LAWSON, D. D.: The protective effect of inhalation of oxygen at 2 atmospheres absolute pressure in acute coronary occlusion. *Surg. Gynec. Obstet., 114:*320, 1962.

25. TRAPP, W. G., AND CREIGHTON, R.: Experimental studies of increased atmospheric pressure on myocardial ischaemia after coronary ligation. *J. Thorac. Cardiov. Surg., 47:*687, 1964.

26. TRAPP, W. G., AND CREIGHTON, R.: Experimental studies of increased oxygen pressure on myocardial ischaemia after coronary ligation. Ref. 3 above, p. 100.

27. VAN ELK, J., AND TRIPPEL, O. H.: Ventricular fibrillation following coronary occlusion in the dog heart and the possible protective effect of high pressure oxygen. Ref. 3 above, p. 116.

12

Shock

CELLULAR HYPOXIA IS THE devastating concomitant of shock.[7,11] The benefits of oxygen administration toward combating its consequences have been long recognized.[4] In states of serious impairment of perfusion, oxygen therapy at atmospheric pressure may prove inadequate in relieving hypoxia for lack of provision of an adequate supply of the gas. Irreversibility is considered likely if the resulting oxygen debt exceeds about 120 ml/kg. Whatever the extent of the debt in shock, hyperoxygenation of arterial blood should be more effective in relieving it than usual methods of oxygen therapy.

Although an early interest in the use of H.O. in the treatment of shock was manifested abroad,[5] the researches of Cowley and his associates[1-3,6-9,12] at the University of Maryland have been outstanding. Their particular interest has been in the treatment of hemorrhagic shock in dogs. Utilizing oxygen at 3 atmospheres absolute, survival rate was elevated from 17 per cent in the control group breathing air to 74 per cent in those treated with H.O. after bleeding and before reinfusion. Heart rate decreased and blood pressure rose in the animals during H.O. Oxygen saturation of arterial blood rose and the partial pressure of carbon dioxide fell after exposure to H.O. Muscle oxygen tension rose from a low of 10 mm Hg to a stable level of 50 mm Hg. Some convulsive evidence of oxygen toxicity was encountered. Tris-(hydroxymethyl) aminomethane (THAM) was not effective in lowering mortality.

Experiments with rats exposed to tumbling shock in a Noble-Collip drum were likewise encouraging in the reduction of mortality from 60 per cent in controls to 20 per cent in those animals transferred to a hyperbaric chamber and exposed to oxygen at 3 atmospheres absolute for a period of two hours following drumming.

Results obtained in studies[7,10] with bacteremic shock have been most disappointing. Cowley and coworkers[7] feel that although hypoxia was relieved in dogs whose peritoneal cavities were contaminated with a saline suspension of feces, the oxygen concentration within the cavities may have been elevated only sufficiently to favorably affect the growth of bacteria. The resulting endotoxin was considered to have interfered with cellular metabolism so that adverse biochemical changes in the animals treated with H.O. were more severe than those in the controls. Incision and direct exposure of the peritoneal cavity to oxygen at elevated partial pressures has been suggested as being more beneficial.

The author is unaware of the clinical use of H.O. in the treatment of hemorrhagic, traumatic or bacterial shock. Indirectly, the benefits of H.O. reported in the surgical management of congenital cardiac defects, in the treatment of poisonings with carbon monoxide and barbiturates, and in the control of the spread of gas gangrene, are probably somewhat related to salutary effects upon existing shock states or to their prevention. These applications are discussed elsewhere.

References

1. ATTAR, S., ESMOND, W. G., BLAIR, E., AND COWLEY, R. A.: Experimental aspects of the use of hyperbaric oxygen in hemorrhagic shock. *Amer. Surg., 30:*243, 1964.

2. ATTAR, S., ESMOND, W. G., AND COWLEY, R. A.: Hyperbaric oxygenation in vascular collapse. *J. Thorac. Cardiov. Surg., 44:* 759, 1962.

3. BLAIR, E., *et al.*: Effect of hyperbaric oxygenation (OHP) on bacteremic shock. *Circulation, 29:*135, 1964.

4. BOOTHBY, W. M., MAYO, C. E., AND LOVELACE, W. R.: One hundred per cent oxygen: Indications for its use and methods of its administration. *J.A.M.A., 113:*477, 1939.

5. BURNET, W.: Treatment of shock by O_2 under pressure. *Scot. Med. J., 4:*535, 1959.

6. COWLEY, R. A.: Hyperbaric oxygenation in hypoxic shock states. *Dis. Chest, 46:*112, 1964.

7. COWLEY, R. A., ATTAR, S., BLAIR, E., ESMOND, W. G., MICHAELIS, M., AND OLLODART, R.: Prevention and treatment of shock by hyperbaric oxygenation. *Ann. N.Y. Acad. Sci., 117:*673, 1965.

8. COWLEY, R. A., ATTAR, S., ESMOND, W. G., BLAIR, E., AND HAW-

THORNE, I.: Electrocardiographic and biochemical study in hemorrhagic shock in dogs treated with hyperbaric oxygenation. *Circulation, 27:*670, 1963.

9. ESMOND, W. G., ATTAR, S., AND COWLEY, R. A.: Hyperbaric oxygenation in experimental hemorrhagic shock: Experimental chamber design and operation. *Trans. Amer. Soc. Artif. Intern. Organs, 8:*384, 1962.

10. EVANS, W. E., *et al.:* The use of hyperbaric oxygen in the treatment of endotoxin shock. *Surgery, 56:*184, 1964.

11. HYPERBARIC OXYGENATION: Potentialities and Problems. Report of the Ad Hoc Committee on Hyperbaric Oxygenation, Committee on Shock, Division of Medical Sciences, National Academy of Sciences, National Research Council, Washington, 1963.

12. MOULTON, G. H., ESMOND, W. G., AND MICHAELIS, M.: Effect of hyperbaric oxygenation on Noble-Collip drum shock in the rat. *Bull. Sch. Med. Univ. Maryland, 47:*42, 1962.

13

Hyaline Membrane Disease

THIS PULMONARY AFFLICTION of the newborn, characterized by respiratory distress and hypoxia, would suggest the likelihood of favorable response to H.O. Accordingly, Hutchison and his associates[3] conducted a series of clinical trials which led to a gratifying clinical impression of a significant reduction of mortality. The report attracted favorable comment.[5] Subsequently, with extension of their clinical experience in the treatment of the disease, impressions[1] changed to disappointment due to the fact that whereas H.O. does relieve hypoxia, it does not correct respiratory acidosis. Indeed, in addition to having nothing to offer in the treatment of hyaline membrane disease, H.O. is suspected of contributing a detrimental effect.

Laboratory evidence has been reported by Shanklin and Berman[4] which is consistent with the suspicion of a possible detrimental effect. Their studies indicated that bilateral cervical vagotomy produced in newborn rabbits a histopathologic condition similar to that of hyaline membrane disease in infants. H.O. exerted a synergistic effect in the production of pathologic changes in such animals.

Upon the basis of available evidence, the use of H.O. in the treatment of hyaline membrane disease seems destined for abandonment.

References

1. HUTCHISON, J. H.: Comments in *Ann. N.Y. Acad. Sci., 117:*706 and 722, 1965.
2. HUTCHISON, J. H., KERR, M. M., DOUGLAS, T. A., INALL, J. A., AND CROSBIE, J. C.: A therapeutic trial in 100 cases of the respiratory distress syndrome of the newborn. *Pediatrics, 33:*956, 1964.
3. HUTCHISON, J. H., KERR, M. M., MCPHAIL, F. M., DOUGLAS, T. A., SMITH, G., NORMAN, J. N., AND BATES, E. H.: Studies in the treatment of the pulmonary syndrome of the newborn. *Lancet,* 2:465, 1962.

4. SHANKLIN, D. R., AND BERMAN, P. A.: The influence of hyperbaric oxygen on hyaline membrane disease in newborn rabbits. *Southern Med. J.*, *56*:1443, 1963.

5. TRAPP, W. G.: The therapeutic use of high-pressure oxygen. *Canad. Med. Ass. J.*, *88*:356, 1963.

14

Hyperbaric Anesthesia

HYPERBARIC INHALATION ANESTHESIA may or may not provide H.O. concomitantly. The concept was conceived by Bert[2] as a means for extending the potentiality of a weak anesthetic. He purported to provide surgical anesthesia without hypoxia using a mixture of 5/6 nitrous oxide and 1/6 oxygen at a pressure of 6/5 atmospheres absolute. The technique was never clinically popular probably for lack of a specific indication.

In 1927, Brown and his associates[5] criticized Bert's claims and further concluded from their own experiments that the depressant effect of nitrous oxide is inevitably associated with hypoxemia. This latter conclusion is not consistent with observations during modern anesthesia with nitrous oxide at atmospheric pressure nor with the findings of Faulconer and coworkers [10] who produced light surgical anesthesia with a 50:50 mixture of the gas with oxygen at 2 atmospheres absolute without significant alteration in the oxygen saturation of arterial blood.

Subsequently, the hyperbaric technique was employed by Pittinger and associates[19] to produce profound anesthesia with xenon, a gas comparable in potency to nitrous oxide. With adequately controlled ventilation, the saturation of hemoglobin with oxygen was maintained even though the partial pressure of the gas was 200 mm Hg while that of xenon approached 3 atmospheres absolute. Theoretically the same should be possible with nitrous oxide. Obviously, the simultaneous achievement of profound nitrous oxide anesthesia and H.O. would require greater chamber pressures than if the same partial pressure of oxygen were provided during anesthesia with a potent agent.

In spite of Tindal's reference[24] to anesthesia by the method of Bert as "the perfect anaesthetic," the validity of the appellation requires proof. There is evidence suggesting that hyperbaric nitrous oxide may not be inocuous. Headache, malaise, gastric distress and psychic depression have occurred after it.[9] The depression[11,14] of hemopoiesis in bone marrow after prolonged nitrous oxide administration in lesser than anesthetizing concentrations suggests the possibility of augmentation of this effect with hyperbaric tensions of the gas. In our own experience,[19] one of the animals that had well tolerated profound xenon anesthesia succumbed during an attempt to repeat the experiment later the same day with nitrous oxide. It should be emphasized that these evidences are only suggestive. They should not be construed to contra-indicate the use of nitrous oxide in hyperbaric procedures, especially if its partial pressure does not exceed that commonly employed in anesthesia. Under the latter condition of its use in H.O., nitrous oxide should present no particular hazard of decompression sickness or diffusion anoxia during appropriate decompression. A purposeful use of nitrous oxide at hyperbaric tensions might be for reducing white cell count in leukemia. Whether such an effect would significantly alter morbidity or mortality is unknown.

In the current revivification of interest in hyperbaric anesthesia,[6,15-18,20-23] emphasis is upon H.O. wherein the hazards of fire and explosion commonly associated with ordinary anesthesia are greatly enhanced. All flammable agents are precluded from use. Cyclopropane, ethylene and the various ethers, except methoxyflurane, are thereby excluded from consideration. In addition to the latter drug, halothane, chloroform and nitrous oxide are left as possibilities. Halothane has probably been most widely used in mixtures with oxygen. Smith and coworkers[22,23] prefer a nitrous oxide and oxygen combination with the partial pressure of the anesthetic at only about 0.3 atmospheres absolute when total pressure is 3 atmospheres absolute. As an adjunct he employs a non-depolarizing, muscle relaxant. Sanger and associates[21] reported the use of intravenous barbiturates for radiotherapy. The usual advantages of inhalation over intravenous techniques in surgery should apply to hyperbaric anesthesia unless future findings indicate otherwise.

The selection of anesthetics for use in H.O. is largely emperical, being attended by unsolved pharmacologic problems. Uncertainty exists concerning their effects upon cortical and total cerebral blood flow as influenced by vasodilatory or vasoconstricting action. The matter is complicated by the impact of carbon dioxide and/or oxygen; the tensions of these are subject to variation with ventilation. What little is known pertains to normal human beings and animals studied at atmospheric pressure. Even if these problems were settled, the question remains whether or not the selection of a particular agent favoring dilation of vessels and a high perfusion of cerebral tissues with oxygen is desirable. Conceivably, high oxygen perfusion would favor toxicity; excessive vasoconstriction might cause hypoxia.

Anesthetics considered non-flammable under ordinary conditions of usage may not be so when administered during H.O. According to Cecil Gray,[3] the findings of Imperial Chemical Industries, Ltd., relative to halothane indicate that this agent with oxygen up to 3 atmospheres absolute is safe. At this pressure, concentrations of halothane above 2 per cent exposed to high energy sources can burn. Most important was the observation that under hyperbaric conditions any mixtures of nitrous oxide and oxygen with halothane can burn and hence should be avoided. The author is unaware of data pertaining to the flammability of methoxyflurane and chloroform under hyperbaric conditions.

Other precautionary measures against fire and explosion have been advised.[3,4,7] Rubber, neoprene and plastic anesthetic equipment unless proved otherwise should be considered as potentially dangerous. Replacement of rubber and neoprene with less flammable but conductive silicone has been recommended. Flameproofed materials for apparel and drapes are available. Oils, greases, lubricants and flammable hydraulic fluid for operating tables should be eliminated or replaced with non-flammable substances. The use of cautery and diathermy are precluded. The extent of permissible usage of electronic monitoring devices is questionable. E.K.G. and E.E.G. monitoring have been employed. The former may be particularly helpful because of the interference with auscultory monitoring of heart sounds caused by the elevated noise level within chambers; the latter has been suggested [16] as reasonable for detection of aberrant activity of the brain due to oxygen toxicity since the effect of muscle relaxants may mask other evidences of convulsion.

The functioning of anesthetic equipment and adjunctive instruments may be altered under hyperbaric conditions. Vaporizers such as the Fluotec should theoretically be usable at the same dial settings during hyperbaric operation as at normal pressure. This generalization assumes unchanged efficiency at all settings. The number of molecules released from the surface of a volatile liquid is determined by temperature; pressure effects are inconsequential in this regard. At 3 atmospheres absolute, for instance, the number of vehicular molecules trebles while that of the volatile agent remains unchanged. Percentage of the agent in the emerging flow from the vaporizer is one third of what it would be at atmospheric pressure. However, since total pressure has trebled, so would the partial pressure of the anesthetic. Hence the latter is similar at atmospheric pressure and at 3 atmospheres absolute; theoretically it should remain so at all elevations of pressure. Since anesthetic effect is a function of partial pressure rather than percentage composition, it should be no different at elevated pressures than under ordinary circumstances, provided physiologic conditions are unchanged by other drugs or physical influences.

However, in a study of the composition of gases emerging from two Fluotec vaporizers, McDowall[16] found the above to hold for halothane, except at dial settings below 2 per cent where the partial pressure of the agent at 2 atmospheres absolute was considerably in excess of that at atmospheric pressure. The reason for the discrepancy is not known. It is possibly related to pressure effects upon relative efficiency of functioning of the vaporizers at different dial settings. No clinical difficulties were reported by Smith and his associates[22,23] in their use of a Fluotec vaporizer at a setting between 0.5 per cent and 1.5 per cent assuming a constancy of partial pressure of halothane vapor, regardless of pressure changes.

McDowall also studied[16] the functioning of rotameters and a Wright respirometer at 2 atmospheres absolute and found both in error. The actual delivery of a gas was less by about 29 per cent than the indicated reading in two flowmeters tested. According to his equation provided for the approximate correction of this error, actual flow rate at an elevated pressure equals the indicated flow at that pressure multiplied by the square root of the ratio between the density of the gas at the pressure of original calibration of the rotameter and its density at the elevated pressure. Accordingly, at 2 atmospheres absolute, actual flow rate should equal the indicated flow rate multiplied by the square root of one-half. Although not tested at other pressures, the correction factor is presumed to apply. In determinations of minute volume with the Wright respirometer, indicated values were reduced by 20 per cent.

Smith and coworkers[22,23] reported marked discrepancies between the actual and indicated flow rates of oxygen and nitrous oxide measured in uncompensated McKesson gauges. With the flow meter for oxygen set at 1 l/min., actual flow at 3 atmospheres absolute was only 0.48 l/min. They suggested the calibration of all gauges at various pressures of usage.

In our experiments,[19] two other difficulties were encountered. One was the erratic functioning of a pH meter at hyperbaric pressure. The other pertained to the decreased flow of gas from a high pressure cylinder to which a reducing valve had been attached and adjusted at about 60 psi. As the pressure within the chamber rose, it increasingly opposed that of the emerging gas so that flow decreased appreciably.

As previously reported,[18] the quality of drugs used in anesthesia deserves particular attention when employed at hyperbaric partial pressures. Volatile impurities of a noxious character in gases employed at partial pressures exceeding those used at atmospheric conditions would be increasingly harmful since they too would be administered at elevated partial pressures. High quality compressed gas should be procured from reputable manufacturers and distributors. Dangerous impurities in nitrous oxide have recently been reported.[12,13]

Deterioration of volatile agents upon exposure to heat, light, oxygen, moisture and some metals is known to occur. The formation of 2,3 dichloro 1,1,1,4,4,4 hexafluoro butene-2 through the reaction between halothane, oxygen and copper as reported[8] has doubtful clinical significance under recommended conditions of usage of vaporizers at atmospheric pressure. However, chemical reactions of this nature which are dependent upon oxygen would be expected to accelerate upon hyperoxygenation. A glance at the chemical structures of other halogenated compounds suggests the possibility of their yielding products which might be toxic.

The matter deserves investigation under conditions of hyper-oxygenation. The recommended practice of frequent, periodic emptying of vaporizers, cleansing and refilling with uncontaminated drug would warrant added attention in hyperbaric usage.

The restricted space within hyperbaric chambers even though ventilated, precludes the exhaustion of appreciable quantities of anesthetic gases and vapors within it. It is recommended that these be exhausted through a tube to the outside of the chamber.

The avoidance of serious errors in chemical determinations of blood gases deserves attention. The attendant problems and their management are beyond the scope of this presentation.

Dangers of concern to anesthesiologists may lurk insidiously. In 1940, Behnke[1] suggested from experimental studies of healthy naval personnel that up to half of a civilian population might be unable to accommodate to more than fractional increases in pressure. Reference was to discomfort due to obstructed eustachian tubes or sinuses and to the possibility of rupture of tympanic membranes. Since swallowing or some other maneuver may be necessary to equilibrate pressures on opposite sides of the tympanic membrane, the question arises as to whether anesthesia should be induced before pressurization of the chamber. A trial test of the unanesthetized subject may avoid difficulties; bilateral myringatomies have been advised to avert trouble. The anesthesiologist himself may be unable to participate in hyperbaric therapy involving his presence within a pressurized chamber. If a regular participant, he deserves the periodic physical examination including appropriate x-ray examinations recommended for avoidance and detection of dangerous conditions.

Cuffs around endotracheal tubes which are properly inflated at atmospheric pressure will tend to decrease in size at elevated pressure. It is conceivable that the ensuing leaks may lead to hypoventilation of the patient. Attention to the proper degree of inflation at elevated pressures is necessary. The opposite phenomenon occurs during decompression. Expansion of the volume of gas within the cuff during decompression may lead to rupture of the trachea! Failure to unclamp intra-pleural tubes during decompression could result in tension pneumothorax.

The sedentary habits of some anesthesiologists, especially the more corpulent ones, may present an occupational hazard in hyperbaric practice. Lack of muscular exertion during decompression has been considered the cause of decompression symptoms presumed associated with post-decompression release of dissolved gases from ischemic tissues of the gluteal region! Relief of ischemia in that area by muscular activity during decompression should minimize the risk.

As stated in the chapter on physiologic considerations, the benefits of H.O. are assumed to proceed from the elevation of oxygen tensions in body tissues. The process implies the reflection of alveolar partial pressures of the gas in arterial blood and from there to tissues. For various reasons, discrepancies between alveolar and arterial tensions of oxygen do occur. Such have been reported[16], suggesting a R-L intrapulmonary shunting mechanism considered the result of progressive alveolar collapse due to the anesthetic effect, since the same condition was not observed in unanesthetized subjects. Additional investigation of the potentiality of the various anesthetics in this respect is indicated. Also implied is the need for rapid and reliable methods of oxygen determination in blood and tissues to verify the presumption of hyperoxygenation. Appropriate equipment for reliable, continuous monitoring of this parameter is wanting.

An analogous situation pertains to the need for clarification of the combined effects of H.O. and the various anesthetic drugs upon circulation in general, and in specific areas of particular concern such as the brain and other vital organs. Conceivably, vasoconstriction combined with decreased cardiac output, or either effect singly, might result in considerably lesser tissue oxygenation than that presumed from the tension of the gas in arterial blood and hence oppose the objective of H.O.

In the interests of promoting the development of H.O. and the safety of all concerned with it, the experiences of anesthesiologists should be made available through publication and participation in discussions of the subject. In view of its experimental status, cautious progress involving appropriate forethought and animal experimentation as precedents to clinical application are indicated. Because of uncertainties associated with H.O., particularly close observations of the clinical responses of patients to anesthesia are important.

References

1. BEHNKE, A. R.: High atmospheric pressure. *Ann. Intern. Med., 13:* 2217, 1940.
2. BERT, P.: Sur la possibilité de 'obtenir, a'l'aide due protoxyde d'azote, une insensibilité de longue dureé, et sur l'innocuité de cet anesthesique. *Acad. Sci. (Paris), 87:*728, 1878. English release in: *Med. Press, 27:*99, 1879.
3. BOND, G.: Panel discussion on "safety considerations." *Ann. N.Y. Acad. Sci., 117:*828, 1965.
4. BROWN, O. W. J., AND SMITH, W. W.: General safety features in chamber design and operation. *Ann. N. Y. Acad. Sci., 117:*801, 1965.
5. BROWN, W. E., LUCAS, G. H. W., AND HENDERSON, V. E.: The anesthetic value of nitrous oxide under pressure. *J. Pharmacol. Exp. Ther., 31:*269, 1927.
6. CASS, N. M.: Anesthesia for barotherapy. *J. Coll. Radiol. Aust., 6:* 101, 1962.
7. CLAMANN, H. G.: Fire hazards. *Ann. N.Y. Acad. Sci., 117:*814, 1965.
8. COHEN, N. E., BELLVILLE, J. W., BUDZIKIEWICZ, H., AND WILLIAMS, D.: Impurity in halothane anesthetic. *Science, 141:*899, 1963.
9. FAULCONER, A.: Personal communication.
10. FAULCONER, A., PENDER, J. W., AND BICKFORD, R. G.: The influence of partial pressure of nitrous oxide on the depth of anesthesia and the electro-encephalogram in man. *Anesthesiology, 10:* 601, 1949.
11. GREEN, C. D., AND EASTWOOD, D. W.: Effects of nitrous oxide inhalation on hemopoiesis in rats. *Anesthesiology, 24:*341, 1963.
12. HAGELSTEN, J.: Impurities in nitrous oxide with special reference to carbon monoxide. *Ugeskr Laeg., 125:*237, 1963.
13. HAMELBERG, W., MAHAFFEY, J. S., AND BOND, W. E.: Nitrous oxide impurities: A case report. *Anesth. Analg., 40:*408, 1961.
14. LASSEN, H. C. A., HENRICKSEN, E., NEUKIRCH, R., AND KRISTENSEN, H. S.: Treatment of tetanus, severe bone marrow depression after prolonged nitrous oxide anesthesia. *Lancet, 270:*527, 1956.
15. LANPHIER, E. H.: Special requirements of gas administration and physiological measurement in hyperbaric procedures. *Ann. N.Y. Acad. Sci., 117:*824, 1965.

16. McDowall, D. G.: Anaesthesia in a pressure chamber. *Anaesthesia, 19:*321, 1964.

17. Pinkerton, H. H.: The scope of a pressure chamber in surgery and anaesthesia. *Canad. Anaesth. Soc. J., 9:*389, 1962.

18. Pittinger, C. B.: Considerations of hyperbaric inhalation anesthesia. *Southern Med. J., 57:*395, 1964.

19. Pittinger, C. B., Faulconer, A., Knott, J. R., Pender, J. W., Morris, L. E., and Bickford, R. G.: Electro-encephalographic and other observations in monkeys during xenon anesthesia at elevated pressures. *Anesthesiology, 16:*551, 1955.

20. Rendell-Baker, L., and Jacobson, J. H.: The present status and future possibilities of hyperbaric oxygen therapy. *Anesth. Analg., 43:*520, 1964.

21. Sanger, C., Churchill-Davidson, I., and Thomlinson, R. H.: Anesthesia for radiotherapy under high pressure oxygen. *Brit. J. Anaesth., 27:*436, 1955.

22. Smith, R. M.: Anesthesia during hyperbaric oxygenation. *Ann. N.Y. Acad. Sci., 117:*768, 1965.

23. Smith, R. M., Crocker, D., and Adams, J.: Anesthetic management of patients during surgery under hyperbaric oxygenation. *Anesth. Analg., 43:*766, 1964.

24. Tindal, A.: The perfect anaesthetic - anaesthesia by the method of Paul Bert. *Surgo, 7:*1, 1941.

15

Safety Considerations

A CONCOMITANT OF therapeutic endeavors is the iatrogenic risk assumed by the patient. Hyperbaric therapy offers no exception; it differs from most forms of therapy in that the enhanced hazards of hyperbaricity are largely shared by attendants with the patient inside the pressure chamber. They are, however, not identical.

The possibility of the patient suffering the consequences of oxygen toxicity has been discussed. A small number of convulsions, the Paul Bert effect, have been reported; fortunately serious sequelae apparently have not resulted. A single death from pulmonary complications highly suspected of being the Lorrain Smith effect has been reported[1] concerning a patient who convulsed during H.O. and then was continually exposed to oxygen at atmospheric pressure. Assuming adequate ventilation of the chamber, other occupants should not be endangered by oxygen toxicity.

Hazards associated with hyperbaric anesthesia have been discussed in the chapter devoted to the subject. The paucity of information regarding possible altered drug effects and their masking by anesthesia deserves serious consideration and warrants close observation of the patient. Prophylactic myringotomies prior to hyperbaric anesthesia have been advised to avert rupture of tympanic membranes. The same procedure has been suggested for infants or others unable to communicate even though unanesthetized during H.O.

The length of hyperbaric exposure of patients during surgery may be minimized[5] by performance of considerable portions of the procedure before elevation of chamber pressure.

Caution is necessary to relieve pressure from expanding gas within body cavities during decompression. Attention has been directed to the possibility of rupture of the trachea due to increased pressure within cuffs on endotracheal tubes and of the development of pneumothorax or pneumoperitoneum if these cavities are unvented. Distention of the stomach is a likely possibility and should be relieved with a gastric tube. Consideration has been given to the inadvertent production of pneumoperitoneum in females through pressure effects transmitted through fallopian tubes; such is not known to have occurred.

Lack of attention to intravenous infusions during hyperbaric therapy may lead to serious results especially when fluids are contained in bottles. Excessive rate of infusion or air embolism could occur during decompression. Smith and associates[5] advise the use of plastic containers and the clamping of infusion tubes even with these, during both compression and decompression procedures.

Decompression sickness and nitrogen narcosis are hazards more likely to be suffered by attendants breathing pressurized air rather than oxygen. Both have been discussed previously. Although relatively protected because of the inhalation of oxygen which is metabolized, the patient could be indirectly affected by afflictions of his attendants.

Indisputable evidence has been presented[1] that nitrogen narcosis may cause serious impairment of judgment and manual dexterity in persons breathing air at 6 atmospheres absolute. Euphoria has been reported by individuals compressed in air at 3 atmospheres absolute. The critical issue concerns the capabilities of those performing intricate tasks within chambers at prevailing pressures of usage or higher. The seriousness of the problem suggests the possible need at higher pressures for a director of affairs within the chamber, who is equipped to breathe a mixture of non-narcotic gases such as one of helium and oxygen.

Fire and explosion are hazards potentially threatening all occupants of pressurized chambers. The fearsome aspect relates to inescapability, except to a contiguous chamber at similar pressure, since sudden exposure to reduced pressure would result in mass casualties from decompression sickness, and traumatic air embolism resulting from rupture of the lungs. Strict precautions aimed toward prevention of fire indicated the need for elimination of flammable substances and ignition sources where ever possible.

Industrial and military interests in combustion and hazards associated with it have long existed. Unfortunately little investigative work relates to hyperbaric conditions. One is impressed by Clamann[3] of the complexity of combustion and factors influencing it. Among the latter are percentage of oxygen in the atmosphere, its partial pressure as a pure gas or in mixtures, the nature of other gases present, the characteristics of combustible substances, temperature and catalysts. Except for the fact that the danger of combustion increases in relation to the possibilities of collision between molecules of oxygen and those of flammable gases or vapors, it seems unsafe to extrapolate limits of safety from available experimental data. What is known regarding the quenching properties of gases such as nitrogen and helium at atmospheric pressure may not pertain to all hyperbaric conditions.

Lanphier[4] has expressed concern of fire hazard from the possible implosion of vacuum tubes in electrical or electronic equipment and from sparks caused by switches and contacts. Equipment which is explosion-proof at atmospheric pressure may not be safe upon exposure to high pressure, especially in the presence of elevated oxygen tensions.

Bond[1] has suggested the feasibility of maintaining oxygen concentrations within chambers at 10 per cent or less as a means for decreasing fire hazards. Human beings have been subjected continually for twelve days to a pressure exceeding 6 atmospheres absolute in an atmospheres with an oxygen concentration of 3.5 per cent. Under such conditions matches would not light.

Brief comments regarding safety in hyperbaric therapy are scattered through publications of chamber manufacturers and users. Brown and Smith,[2] however, have provided a comprehensive treatment of precautions in relation to their installation at Duke University.

The following collected items refer to precautionary measures presented for consideration rather than as directives. It is realized that subsequent researches may indicate the inadequacy of some of the suggestions and lead to superior alternatives.

a) Use of professionally designed hyperbaric facilities which have been safety-coded according to standards of the American Society of Mechanical Engineers, rather than do-it-yourself, improvised chambers.

b)　　Provision of ungrounded electrical power with an isolation transformer and alarm system to notify of grounding.

c)　　Utilization of electrical cables insulated with mineral rather than organic coverings, and non-sparking electrical switches, receptacles and lights.

d)　　Minimization of the number of electronic devices inside the chamber and provision of pressure-proof housings where necessary.

e)　　Substitution of pneumatic or hydraulic motors for electrical ones.

f)　　Quenching with nitrogen or other suitable gas of electrical equipment which may spark.

g)　　Substitution of flammable greases, oils and hydraulic fluids with suitable silicone or fluorinated derivatives.

h)　　Use of fire-proofed paints, garments and drapes.

i)　　Isolation of defibrillators from ground to avoid burning due to arcing across EKG, EEG and transducer grounds or operating table.

j)　　Venting of anesthetic or other noxious gases directly to the outside of the chamber and insurance of adequate air conditioning to avoid accumulation of dangerous levels of oxygen or fumes.

k)　　Atomized humidification rather than that derived from steam.

l)　　Heating and cooling of chambers with hot water rather than steam and chilled water rather than freon or other refrigerant gases.

m)　　Use of water or even sand rather than carbon dioxide or carbon tetrachloride for fire extinguishers; ceiling-mounted inundating sprays controllable from inside or outside are considered a desirable feature.

n)　　Provision of emergency air and power supplies.

o)　　Maintenance of an emergency air line and adequate numbers of masks to serve all persons in the chamber in case of fire, smoke or fumes.

p)　　Screening of patients and attendants through appropriate medical examinations including x-ray and hematological studies, conducted periodically for attendants who are repeatedly exposed to hyperbaric conditions.

q)   Checking of instruments routinely prior to pressurizing chambers.

r)   Selection of qualified personnel for management of the control panel outside of chamber.

s)   Use of the least pressure and shortest periods of pressurization consistent with needs.

t)   Prior to activation of a facility for clinical use, scheduling of a practice performance to insure consideration of all needs.

u)   Constant observation and/or monitoring of the patient for development of untoward conditions.

v)   Consideration of the need for deviating from established rates of decompression in favor of slower ones suggested by the condition of patients, especially the seriously debilitated, elderly and emphysematous ones.

w)   Acquaintance of attendants with the particular hazards of oxygen toxicity, nitrogen narcosis, decompression sickness and hyperbaric anesthesia.

x)   Restriction of the use of hyperbaric therapy to those conditions for which a scientific rationale for treatment has been established.

The subject of safety undoubtedly will deserve increasing emphasis in the future. Such will be indicated to offset dangers associated with expanding use of hyperbaric equipment. It would seem advisable to delegate administrative authority for the clinical application of H.O. to a responsible physician. The medical and legal implications of unrestricted usage by enthusiastic but unqualified personnel would be prohibitive. Professional qualifications should include competency in the recognition and treatment of medical emergencies that might arise during hyperbaric therapy.

References

1. BOND, G.: Chairman: Panel discussion: Safety considerations. *N.Y. Acad. Sci., 117*:814, 1965.
2. BROWN, I. W., AND SMITH, W. W.: General safety features in chamber design and operation. *Ann. N.Y. Acad. Sci., 117*:801, 1965.
3. CLAMANN, H. G.: Fire hazards. *Ann. N.Y. Acad. Sci., 117*:814, 1965.
4. LANPHIER, E. H.: Special requirements of gas administration and

physiological measurement in hyperbaric procedures. *Ann. N.Y. Acad. Sci., 117:*824, 1965.

5. SMITH, R. M., CROCKER, D., AND ADAMS, J. G.: Anesthetic management of patients during surgery under hyperbaric oxygenation. *Anesth. Analg., 43:*766, 1964.

16

Status of Hyperbaric Oxygenation

THE ACCOMPLISHMENTS OF hyperbaric research and its clinical applications during the past decade have stimulated widespread interest in H.O. Consequently, numerous individuals including basic scientists, clinicians, directors of medical centers and biologic institutions, and hospital administrators are deliberating the initiation of programs of hyperbaric research or therapy in their institutions. As an aid in such deliberations, a concept of the current status of H.O. is offered for consideration. It may be helpful in suggesting a program consistent with reflected needs.

In all aspects, H.O. remains an experimental subject. This consensus is clearly evident from publications and other expressions of opinions by those already engaged in hyperbaric activities. Clinical progress in H.O. thus far does not indicate the termination of the experimental stage but rather the beginning of another phase of it.

Numerous unsolved problems of a basic scientific nature await resolution. What information is available has served to emphasize how little is known and to suggest widespread needs for additional research. Oxygen toxicity, nitrogen narcosis, hyperbaric physiology and pharmacology, and safety measures especially those related to fire hazards require extensive investigation. The presumption of tissue oxygenation commensurate with inhaled or arterial tensions of oxygen is probably not valid in many circumstances. Scientific evaluation and assurance of the optimal benefits of H.O. necessitate development of improved micro-techniques for the continuous determination of oxygen saturation at cellular levels. These and other areas of basic research are essential to progress in hyperbaric therapy and provide broad opportunities to qualified investigators.

Clinical research has been more restricted than that in the basic sciences. Hyperbaric facilities for that purpose are relatively few and costlier. Progress has been slow but definite; it is consistent with the recognized need for a cautious and rational approach to all clinical applications.

Series of cases are slowly being accumulated in the centers of clinical activity. In some instances, applications of H.O., such as that for the correction of congenital cardiac defects in infants, are simultaneously being studied in different locations here and abroad.

A common deficiency characterizes most clinical endeavors. Despite explicit rationales for therapy, the clinical applications of H.O. have been largely empirical. This is not intended as a criticism of those who have pioneered such work. The accumulation of carefully controlled series of clinical cases may be difficult and require a long time. Nevertheless, such a goal is considered necessary if objective evaluation of H.O. is to be achieved. Impressions are mostly subjective. Critical appraisal of clinical accomplishments with H.O. are generally wanting. Comparative, scientific evaluation of the benefits of H.O. in relation to those available through conventional therapeutic regimens is a pressing need in clinical research. Substantiation of the potential benefits of H.O. is important for several reasons: to assure establishment of an appropriate status of H.O. in medicine; to avert its decadence from inappropriate clinical application; to avoid useless expenditures of effort and funds and possible harm to patients.

In addition to establishing current clinical uses of H.O. upon a firmer, scientific basis, the desire to extend its application in new areas is recognized. A rational basis of therapy is essential in all such instances. The harm, which may result from imprudent administration of hyperbaric therapy, is historically documented.

The experimental status of H.O. suggests the prematurity of anticipation of numerous, flourishing centers of hyperbaric therapy in the near future. Clinical research is in its incipient phase. Relatively few clinical uses of H.O. have been demonstrated even in Europe where progress is currently most advanced. Thus far, the best therapeutic indications are confined to diseases of relatively low incidence such as congenital cardiac anomalies, carbon monoxide poisoning and gas gangrene.

The preceding paragraph was not intended to convey disparagement concerning hyperbaric progress or its potentialities.

Contrariwise, it compliments those whose cause in the interest of H.O. is realization of its fullest potentialities through scientific investigation. Such requires prudence and time.

A significant advance in clinical H.O. would be the demonstration of its efficacy in the treatment of one or several diseases of high incidence. The expectation of such an occurrence is reasonable from the apparent interest and basic research related to vascular insufficiency, especially that associated with coronary occlusion. The hyperbaric treatment of shock from various causes is also receiving considerable attention.

The eventual status of H.O. in medicine will be dependent upon the integrity of research, both basic and clinical, sustaining it. De-emphasis of research in favor of clinical empiricism would be inconsistent with the current concept of H.O. and apparent needs to assure progress. The latter will be aided through exchange of pertinent scientific information. Occasionally, a review of the changing status of H.O. will seem indicated. Such a consideration instigated the preparation of this monograph.

Addendum

THE CURRENT INTEREST in H.O. is evident from the rapid expansion of the literature pertaining to it. The following references have come to the attention of the author since preparation of the manuscript. They are appended under appropriate chapter headings to provide as timely a source of selected bibliographic information as is possible.

Historical Development

1. Alvis, H. J.: Hyperbaric medicine today. *Milit. Med., 130:*502, 1965.
2. Hitchcock, C. R., Haglin, J. J., Johnson, F. E., and Haffbauer, F. W.: Hyperbaric medical facility. *Minnesota Med.,* 48:51, 1965.
3. Richter, G., Wernitsch, W., and Frey, R.: Sauerstofftherapie in der Uberdruckkammer. *Deutsch. Med. Wschr., 90:*619, 1965.
4. Saltzman, H. A., and Brown, I. W., Jr.: Hyperbaric medicine. *Ann. Rev. Med., 16:*253, 1965.
5. Sellers, L. M.: The fallibility of the Forrestian principle. *Anesth. Analg.* (Cleveland) , *44:*39, 1965.
6. Severinghaus, J. W.: Annual report of the committee on high oxygen pressure equipment. *Amer. Soc. Anesth. Newsletter, 29:* 1, 1965.
7. Tassel, P. V. Van: A hyperbaric chamber for small animals. *J. Appl. Physiol., 20:*342, 1965.
8. Waters, R. M.: Cunningham's theory revisited. *Anesth. Analg.* (Cleveland) , *44:*469, 1965.

Physiologic Considerations

1. Anderson, B., Jr., Heyman, A., Whalen, R. E., and Saltzman, H.: Visual and cerebral vascular phenomena after decompression from hyperbaric environment. *Neurology (Minneap.), 15:*269, 1965.
2. Gerber, C., *et al.:* Effect of hyperbaric oxygenation on muscle blood flow during reactive hyperemia. *Clin. Res., 13:*59, 1965.
3. Jamieson, D., and Van Den Brenk, H. A. S.: Electrode size and

tissue pO_2 measurement in rats exposed to air or high pressure oxygen. *J. Appl. Physiol., 20:*514, 1965.

4. Lanius, J. W., *et al.:* Surfactant studies with hyperbaric oxygen. *Clin. Res., 13:*74, 1965.

5. Mottram, R. F.: Effect of hyperbaric oxygen on limb circulation. *Lancet, 1:*602, 1965.

6. Saltzman, H. A., and Hall, F. G.: Tissue oxygenation at increased atmospheric pressures. *Physiol. Physicians, 3:*1, 1965.

7. Weglicki, W. B., Whalen, R. E., and McIntosh, H. D.: Effects of hyperbaric oxygenation on excess lactate production in exercising dogs. *Clin. Res., 13:*222, 1965.

8. Whalen, R. E., Saltzman, H. A., Holloway, D. H., McIntosh, H. D., Sieker, H. O., and Brown, I. W.: Cardiovascular and blood gas responses to hyperbaric oxygenation. *Amer. J. Cardiol., 15:*638, 1965.

9. Yanda, R. L., and Motley, H. L.: Changes in lung volume and spirometric measurements in emphysema patients who have been exposed to hyperbaric pressure levels. *Dis. Chest, 47:*360, 1965.

Oxygen Toxicity

1. Bergofsky, E. H., Wang, M. C. H., Yamaki, T., and Jacobson, J. H.: Tissue oxygen and carbon dioxide tensions during hyperbaric oxygenation. *J.A.M.A., 189:*841, 1964.

2. Chance, B., Jamieson, D., and Coles, H.: Energy-linked pyridine nucleotide reduction: inhibitory effects of hyperbaric oxygen in vitro and in vivo. *Nature, 206:*257, 1965.

3. Eyal, Z., Manax, W. G., Black, J. H., and Lillehei, R. C.: Utilization of chlorpromazine in heart storage and its combined use with hyperbaric oxygen and hypothermia. *Surg. Gynec. Obstet., 120:*1237, 1965.

4. Gillen, H. W.: Neurologic hazards of hyperbaric oxygen exposure. *Dis. Chest, 47:*369, 1965.

5. Heppleston, A. G., and Simnett, J. D.: Tissue reaction to hyperbaric oxygen. *Lancet, 1:*964, 1965.

6. Kydd, G. H.: Observations on acute and chronic oxygen poisoning. *Aerospace Med., 35:*1176, 1964.

7. Mengel, C. E., Kann, H. E., Heyman, A., and Metz, E.: Effects of in vivo hyperoxia on erythrocytes. II. Hemolysis in a human after exposure to oxygen under high pressure. *Blood, 25:*822, 1965.

8. Mengel, C. E., Zirkle, L. G., O'Malley, B. W., and Horton, B. D.: Further studies of the mechanism of in vivo RBC damage by oxygen. *Aerospace Med., 36:*154, 1965.
9. Saltzman, H. A., *et al.:* Retinal vascular response to hyperbaric oxygenation. *J.A.M.A., 191:*290, 1965.
10. Stier, H. A., Halasz, N. A.: Tissue reaction to hyperbaric oxygen. *Lancet, 1:*1121, 1964.
11. Webb, W. R., Lanius, J., Aslomi, A., and Reynolds, R.: Surfactant studies with hyperbaric oxygen. *J.A.M.A., 192:*559, 1965.
12. Wood, J. D., Stackey, N. E., and Watson, W. J.: Pulmonary and central nervous system damage in rats exposed to hyperbaric oxygen and protection therefrom by gamma-aminobutyric acid. *Canad. J. Physiol. Pharm., 43:*405, 1965.
13. Zirkle, L. G., Mengel, C. E., Horton, B. D., and Duffy, E. J.: Studies of oxygen toxicity in the central nervous system. *Aerospace Med., 36:*169, 1965.

Decompression Sickness

1. Goodman, M. W.: Decompression sickness treated with compression to 2-6 atmospheres absolute. Report of fourteen cases, discussions and suggestions for a minimal pressure-oxygen breathing therapeutic profile. *Aerospace Med., 35:*1204, 1964.

Clinical Application: Status of the Literature

1. *Hyperbaric Medicine Newsletter,* Vol. 1., No. 1, Jan., 1965. State University of N. Y. at Buffalo, School of Medicine.

Cancer Therapy

1. Hodge, T. G.: Oxygen's therapeutic value in malignancies. *J. Okla. Med. Ass., 58:*204, 1965.
2. Wildermuth, O.: The case for hyperbaric oxygen radiotherapy. *J.A.M.A., 191:*986, 1965.

Surgery

1. Aldrete, J. S., and Judd, E. S.: Gas gangrene: a complication of elective abdominal surgery. *Arch. Surg. (Chicago), 90:*745, 1965.
2. Almond, C. H., Anido, H., Seaber, A., Young, R., and Mackensie, J. W.: Heart preservation utilizing hyperbaric oxygen and hypothermia. *Amer. Heart J., 69:*425, 1965.
3. Boerema, I.: The use of hyperbaric oxygen. *Amer. Heart J., 69:* 289, 1965.

4. Cross, F. S.: Hybaroxic treatment of experimental intestinal obstruction. *Dis. Chest, 47:*374, 1965.
5. Manax, W. G., Black, J. H., Eyal, Z., Lyons, G. W., and Lillehei, R. C.: Hypothermia and hyperbaria: simple method for whole organ preservation. *J.A.M.A., 192:*755, 1965.
6. Slack, W. K., Thomas, D. A., and Perrins, D.: Hyperbaric oxygenation in chronic osteomyelitis. *Lancet, 1:*1093, 1965.

Anaerobic and Other Infections

1. Caldwell, J.: Effects of high partial pressures of oxygen on fungi and bacteria. *Nature, 206:*321, 1965.
2. Chandler, P. J., *et al.:* The effects of intermittent hyperbaric oxygen therapy on the development of tuberculosis in the rabbit. *Amer. Rev. Resp. Dis., 91:*855, 1965.
3. Glad, R. M., Bouhoutsos, D. E., and Douglas, F. M.: Effect of hyperbaric oxygen therapy and changing surgical concepts of gas gangrene. Four case reports. *Amer. J. Surg., 109:*230, 1965.
4. Ross, R. M. and McAllister, T. A.: Protective action of hyperbaric oxygen in mice with pneumococcal septicaemia. *Lancet, 1:*579, 1965.
5. Smart, J. F., Bobb, J. R. J., and Wasmuth, C. E.: Gas gangrene treated with hyperbaric oxygenation. Report of a case. *Cleveland Clin. Quart., 32:*57, 1956.

Resuscitation: Poisonings, Asphyxia Neonatorum, Cardiac Arrest

1. Goulon, M., Barois, A., Rapin, M., Nouailhat, F., Augustin, P., Hennetier, G., Baguet, J. C., Kuntziger, H., and Breteau, M.: Traitement de l'intoxication oxycarbonee par l'oxygene hyperbare (a propos de 20 observations). *Bull. Soc. Med. Hop. Paris, 116:*649, 1965.
2. James, L. S., and Adamsons, K., Jr.: Respiratory physiology of the fetus and new born infant. *New Eng. J. Med., 271:*1352, 1964.
3. Schwartz, S. I., Breslan, R. C., Kutner, F., and Smith, D.: Effects of drugs and hyperbaric oxygen environment on experimental kerosene pneumonitis. *Dis. Chest, 47:*353, 1965.
4. Skene, W. G., and Norman, J. N.: The effect of hyperbaric oxygen in cyanide poisoning. *Scot. Med. J., 10:*87, 1965.

Cardiovascular Insufficiency

1. Hansen, O. M., and Haxholdt, B. F.: Traumatic vascular insufficiency treated with hyperbaric oxygen. *Danish Med. Bull., 12:* 51, 1965.

2. Heyman, A., Whalen, R. E., and Saltzman, H.: The protective effect of hyperbaric oxygenation in cerebral hypoxia. *Trans. Amer. Neurol. Ass., 89:*59, 1964.

3. Ingvar, D. H., and Lassen, N. A.: Treatment of focal cerebral ischemia with hyperbaric oxygen. Report of 4 cases. *Acta Neurol. Scand., 41:*92, 1965.

4. Kuhn, L. A., Kline, H. J., Wang, M., Yamaki, T., and Jacobson, J. H.: Hemodynamic effects of hyperbaric oxygenation in experimental acute myocardial infarction. *Cir. Res., 16:*499, 1965.

5. Peter, R. H., Entman, M. L., Rau, R. W., Whalen, R. E., and McIntosh, H. D.: Effects of hyperbaric oxygenation on experimental coronary occlusion in pigs. *Clin. Res., 13:*217, 1965.

6. Rapin, M., Goulon, M., Nouailhat, F., Barois, A., Got, C., Hennetier, G., and Levy-Alcover, M.: Quatre cas d'accident neurologigue precoce post abortum par embolie gazeuse probable, traites par l'oxygene hyperbare. *Bull. Soc. Med. Hop. Paris, 116:*673, 1965.

7. Saltzman, H. A.: Hyperbaric oxygen in cardiovascular disease: potential usages and hazards. *Circulation, 31:*454, 1965.

8. Siegel, W.: Cardiac work capacity following coronary artery occlusion with air, oxygen and hyperbaric oxygen environments. *Texas Rep. Biol. Med., 22:*800, 1964.

9. Trapp, W. G.: Hyperbaric oxygen and cardiac infarction. *Dis. Chest, 47:*367, 1965.

10. Waddell, W. B., Saltzman, H. A., Fuson, R. L., and Harris, J.: Purpura gangrenosa treated with hyperbaric oxygenation. *J.A.M.A., 191:*971, 1965.

11. Yacoub, M. H., and Zeitlin, G. L.: Hyperbaric oxygen in the treatment of the post-operative low-cardiac-output syndrome. *Lancet, 1:*581, 1965.

Shock

1. Elliott, D. P., and Paton, B. C.: Effect of 100 per cent oxygen at 1 and 3 atmospheres on dogs subjected to hemorrhagic hypotension. *Surgery, 57:*401, 1965.

2. Evans, W. E., and Darin, J. C.: The additive effects of low molecular weight dextran in the treatment of endotoxin shock with hyperbaric oxygen. *J. Trauma, 5:*213, 1965.
3. Meyerowitz, B. R.: Present status of hyperbaric oxygenation with some personal observations on its value in tumbling shock and in barbiturate poisoning. *Amer. J. Surg., 109:*611, 1965.
4. Ollodart, R., and Blair, E.: High-pressure oxygen as an adjunct in experimental bacteremic shock. *J.A.M.A., 191:*736, 1965.

Hyperbaric Anesthesia

1. McDowall, D. G.: Observations on hyperbaric oxygenation during anaesthesia. *Proc. Roy. Soc. Med., 58:*325, 1965.
2. Perrimond-Trouchet, R.: Caissons d'oxygenotherapie hyperbare. *Anesth. Analg. (Paris), 21:*310, 1964.
3. Poulsen, H.: Hyperbare Sauerstoff—Therapie. *Anaesthesist, 14:*115, 1965.
4. Richter, G.: Die Uberdruckkammer—Indikation und Gefahren. *Anaesthesist, 14:*97, 1965.
5. Rodenwald, G., Harms, H., and Donhardt, A.: Konstruktion und Anwendung einer Sauerstoff—Uberdruckkammer. *Anaesthesist, 14:*104, 1965.
6. Vermeulen-Cranch, D. M. E.: Anaesthesia in a high pressure chamber. *Proc. Roy. Soc. Med., 58:*319, 1965.
7. Waters, R. M.: Cunningham's theory revisited. *Anesth. Analg. (Cleveland), 44:*469, 1965.

Safety Considerations

1. Anderson, B., Jr., Whalen, R. E., and Saltzman, H. A.: Dysbarism among hyperbaric personnel. *J.A.M.A., 190:*1043, 1964.

Status of Hyperbaric Oxygenation

1. Schraibman, I. G.: The present scope of hyperbaric therapy. *Med. J. Aust., 1:*642, 1965.
2. Whalen, R. E., and McIntosh, H. D.: Hyperbaric oxygenation: potentials and problems. *Amer. Heart. J., 69:*725, 1965.

Author Index

Subject Index